Home Favorites:

An Introduction to the Diversity of Cameroonian Cuisine

Theresia Niba

ISBN 13: 9781636031019
Library of Congress Catalog Card Number: 2021911075

Table of Contents

PART TWO

PART THREE

PRAYER

In the name of the Father, and of the Son, and of the Holy Spirit. AMEN.

Our Heavenly Father we come before you as your children to whom you said seek and you will find and knock, and it will be opened. May you be the unseen reader to this book. Bless and protect all those who have contributed to its success. Into your hands I commit those who will use this book to have the satisfaction they so desire.

May our mother Mary continue to be our Model as she intercedes to her son on our behalf. We ask this through Christ our Lord who lives and reigns with the Holy Spirit, One God for ever and ever. Amen.

In the name of the Father, and of the Son, and of the Holy Spirit. AMEN.

DEDICATION

To my children, Engelbert, Dymphna, Katrina, Maria- Goretti, and my grandchildren Daphne, Gisele, Wynter and Blu-Arie.

ACKNOWLEDGEMENT

To have come out with a book like this is not an easy task. It has been the work of many people putting hands on deck. First and foremost, I wish to thank the almighty God for many blessings of good health He has given me, and the knowledge He has endowed me with to carry out this work.

My heartfelt thanks go to my beloved husband Niba Tafor Fidelis, who encouraged me to go ahead, showed interest in this project from the beginning to the end, giving useful suggestions, and was the first taster.

Many thanks go to my loving family who took the project as a family duty, supporting it financially, morally, physically, and socially, while also joining me in laughter when the sample dishes came out either good or bad. I appreciate the inspiration of writing which came from the Bishop of Buea, and former Director of Maryvale Institute, Bamenda His Lordship Michael Miabesue Bibi when I was a student at the Maryvale Institute of Bamenda. Many thanks go Mrs. Ambe Veronica Ngum Ngu for her supporting role.

My heartfelt gratitude goes to all those who helped me in this great venture to bring my idea into reality. Those who encouraged me in doing one thing or another especially, the tasters, the drivers, the typists, the proofreaders, the market women who taught me local names of herbs and spices, and even introduced new ones to me. Many thanks also go to Asah Julienne, Yufeh Maureen, Che-Bienka Elizabeth Asana, Njefi Jessica, Shu Hasper Numfor, Ambe Henry, Michael Niba, Ngwa Tanji Felix, and Regina Wirkom. There are many people who are not mentioned here but they shall ever be remembered whenever this book is used. All I can say is:

"To God be the glory great things He has done."

FOREWARD

Man's life on earth depends essentially on the food that he eats to sustain his life. Samuel Beckett puts it more strikingly when he says that life is eating and defecating and waiting for death. Whether we like it or not, man toils on earth because he wants to place food on his table to sustain his life till the final bell for eternal sleep tolls. In toiling for our daily bread many people pay scant attention to the food that they eat. In short, the eating habit of many people, the world over is shrouded in total confusion. The families that scratch the earth for a living can barely afford one meal per day. Furthermore, there are other people who have the food to eat but because of job constraints or other obligations in their daily activities they lack time to devote to their meals. Mrs. Niba Theresia with specialist knowledge in food and nutrition tells us how we have to eat the food that we toil for. In the book entitled coffee: Star Culinary Arts Book One to Home Favorites: An Introduction to the Diversity of Cameroonian Cuisine. Mrs. Niba Theresia lays bare the different dishes that we have to eat. In this book the author is emphatic that we should eat like a king in the morning, like a prince in the afternoon and like a beggar in the evening. Put simply, Mrs. Niba means that the first two meals of the day namely: breakfast and lunch should be very rich while supper, the third meal of the day, should be frugal. In a bid to remain healthy, Mrs. Niba stresses in her book, we should pay close attention to the food that we eat. If we care about our meals, we should buy a copy of Mrs. Niba's book to savour its richness in content and the different dishes proposed.

Professor Ndongmanji J. Niba

INTRODUCTION

Home Favorites are three books that give an intensive view of Cameroon cuisine. These books are a fine jewel to be owned by anyone who wishes to prepare indigenous, attractive, tasty, palatable, and nutritious Cameroon dishes. They are practical books and are very good resource books for instructors and students of culinary arts in Technical, Vocational, and Teacher Training colleges. Persons involved in the hospitality industry such as caterers, hotel managers, restaurant chefs, and event planners will love the books and they will serve as handbooks for tourists who will want to understand the eating culture of Cameroon. Young and working mothers will find them a valuable aid to ease and enrich their cooking skills, while reducing the length of time they will spend in the kitchen, and will also be useful to those who are not in the country,

The importance of these books cannot be underestimated. The collection, and choosing of recipes, was based on predetermined criteria such as the availability of the ingredients and costs, ease in the preparation of dishes, duration of cooking, new knowledge, and skills to be learnt, improvement on traditional dishes, introduction of new vegetables and fruits, upgrading of local methods of cooking, a revision of traditional names of ingredients and dishes, and health benefits of the dishes and the Biblical study of foods. The user will be able to prepare balanced meals, serve them properly, view the many attractive pictures of ingredients, and a great variety of finished dishes found in this treasure, all prepared in the author's beautiful kitchen.

If you are a Christian it is good to understand what the Holy Bible says about food. According to the King James Bible Version there are 466 verses talking about bread, 4 on broth, 11 on butter, 5 on cheese, 27 on cooking, 6 on cream, 15 on delicacies, 17 on dough, 452 on drink, 61 on equipment, 614 on family, 78 on flour, 506 on grain, 64 on honey, 78 on hunger, 29 on leaven, 13 on leftover, 26 on loaf, 18 on manna, 19 on meal, 17 on morsel, 1 on pancake, 13 on paste, 67 on provision, 12 on raw, 70 on spices, 9 on stew, 5 on wafer, 44 on yeast, and 1207 on food.

Some healing foods in the Bible are: olive and olive oil (Deuteronomy 6:7-8), pomegranate (Deuteronomy 6:7-8), small fruits (figs, grapes, berries Gen. 3:7, Gen. 9:20), fermented grapes (Song of Solomon 1:2), flax (Proverbs 31:10, 13), sprouted grain bread (Ezekiel 4:9), grains: barley & wheat (Deut. 8:8, John 6:9-13), raw milk, cultured dairy from goats, cows and sheep (Proverbs 27: 27), lamb (Exodus 12:11), bitter herbs (Exodus 12:8), green vegetables, cultured and fermented vegetables, vegetables (Daniel 1:12), raw honey (Proverbs 15:16), fish and fish oil (Lev. 11:9-12), soups and stocks (Judges 6:19), healthy saturated fats (high vitamins, butter, coconut oil.), wild animal foods, seeds (soaked & sprouted), Omega-3 egg, and organ meats. These dishes can be included in the diet for health and longevity, thus most of the dishes in these books have these ingredients.

These books are basic, as well as advanced books, as they can be used at any level of the educational system, because the recipes are short, simple, and easy to read and prepare. Book One has two parts, notes on Cameroon cookery, culinary skills, and and introduction into the hospitality industry, while Book Two has recipes of the Cameroon dishes, in both French and English. Beautiful, computerized pictures of finished dishes by the author are included.

PART ONE

In this part there is an intensive glossary of culinary terms, in both English and French, making it an advantage to speakers of one, or both languages. Culinary herbs and spices in Cameroon cuisine included in the book help in their identification and the correct usage of Cameroon, African, and International spices. Description of Cameroon foods such as the fufu dish, dishes of the tubers, maize, rice, and plantain are included. Vegetables such as amaranth leaves, bitter leaves, nightshades, the African eggplant, the Eru leaf, meat, seafood, poultry products, the Mbongo Tchobi, Domba dishes, nuts and berries, Cameroon buttery fruits, and palmnut jus are explained.

PART TWO

Meal and meal planning, types of meals, mealtimes, and meal courses are included. A six-week daily menu helps young working mothers to prepare nutritious, tasty, and balanced meals for their families, avoiding long hours in the kitchen. Reception menus help in the planning of various dishes for all types of parties. Food presentation makes food attractive to eat, as the saying goes “we first eat with the eyes”. Basic cooking ingredients are described and are available in our local markets and at affordable prices. Beverages, such as locally brewed drinks such as the shaa, culinary skills and Cameroon flour processing are included.

PART THREE

The hospitality industry: Restaurant and Hotel management and Catering.

GLOSSARY OF CULINARY TERMS

DEFINITION OF TERMS

ALLUMETTE: Potatoes cut into pieces the size and shape of matchsticks, 3cm x 3cm x 5cm.

BASTE: This is to spoon liquid or melted fat over food during cooking.

BLANCH: To cook food in boiling water for a brief period of time and then immersing in cold water to stop the cooking. This applies to vegetables so as to reduce their final cooking time, to remove strong flavors, and to whiten them. It can also be done to meat and fish.

BLEND: The gradual and careful mixing of a powder with cold liquid before adding to hot liquid. The combination of different flavors, textures, and colors by mixing them with spoon, beater, or liquidizer to make that which is desired.

BRAISING: A cooking method by which food is browned with fat, then cooked slowly in a covered pot with little moisture at low heat for a period of time. This method combines frying, simmering, and steaming.

BUTTERMILK: A tangy, butter-flecked liquid left over when whole milk has been churned to make butter. It is sold as low-fat or non-fat milk.

CANAPÉ: A small bite-size piece of bread with various toppings such as smoked salmon, foie, gras, caviar, smoked duck breast, ham, etc., which are served as appetizers.

CAPERS: The small buds of a Mediterranean shrub. They are usually pickled in vinegar or dried and salted.

CASSEROLE: Fireproof earthenware or glass dish with lid used for oven cooking of stews etc.

CAYENNE PEPPER: A very hot ground spice derived from Chili peppers.

CHINOISE: A conical strainer or sieve used to strain sauces and soups.

CIDER VINEGAR: Pale golden vinegar with flavor and a crisp tang of apple vinegar.

CLARIFY: A process which uses egg whites to remove fat and sediment.

CONCASSEE: The term used for chopping vegetables coarsely. Blanched, peeled, quartered and de-seeded tomatoes, finely chopped.

CONFECTIONER'S SUGAR: Pure icing sugar.

CONSOMMEE: Clear soup made from richly flavored stock or bouillon that has been clarified, thus known as "clear" or "double" consommé. Cold consommé is often jelly-like.

CREAM: It is a thick white or yellow fatty liquid which arises to the top when milk is left to stand, and which can be eaten as an accompaniment to desserts or used as a cooking ingredient.

CREPES: These are very thin pancakes made from a batter consisting of milk, flour, eggs. They can be plain with a sprinkling of sugar and lemon juice or spread filled with jam or chocolate and served as a dessert. They can be stuffed with vegetables or fillings and served as a savory dish.

DASH: A measuring term referring to a very small amount of seasoning added to food somewhere between 1/16 and a scant 1/8 teaspoon.

DECANT: Gradually pour wine, port, or other liquid from one container into another typically in order to separate out sediment.

DEGLAZE: The process of removing browned small particles of food from the bottom of the pan after sautéing (usually meat). The technique requires the removal of excess fat from the pan using an acid base item as wine.

DICE: To cut food into tiny cubes between 1/8 inch and ¼ inch square.

EMINCER: To cut food into thin slices shorter than julienne. The term is most often used when referring to meats, but it also applies to fruits and vegetables.

EMULSIFY: To bind together two liquid ingredients that normally does not combine smoothly such as water and fat. Mayonnaise and Vinaigrettes are emulsions.

FILLET: To remove the flesh from fish bones in natural section.

FRICASSEE: To cook by braising, usually applied to fowl or rabbit.

FLAMBE: Pouring spirits such as brandy, rum, or grand marnier over food and setting light to it, used with both savory and sweet dishes.

GARNISH: To decorate a savory dish with edibles of ornamental appearance.

GELATINE: A colorless, translucent, brittle, flavorless food derived from collagen obtained from various animal raw materials (connective tissue, bones, sinews etc.)

GLAZE: To brush the surface of the food with a coating of egg, milk, sugar, and water, etc., during or after cooking.

GUACAMOLE: A mixture of fresh avocado, lime or lemon juice, other seasonings frequently made with diced onions, tomatoes, and cilantro.

GREEN ONIONS: A variety of onion harvested immature before the bulb is formed. It is also called scallions or spring onions.

GRILL: A device for cooking food over a charcoal or a gas fire outdoors.

GRILLING: Cooking with intense heat, provided by gas, electricity, or charcoal. Meat, fish, poultry, vegetables, and some fruit can be cooked this way.

HABANERO CHILI: Small, lantern-shaped green or ripened red chilis measuring 5cm in length and up to 4.5cm wide.

HALF-AND-HALF: A commercial dairy product that is half milk and half light cream.

HEAVY CREAM (WHIPPING CREAM): A rich dairy product with a butter fat content of at least 36%, also known as double cream.

HOLLANDAISE SAUCE: A smooth, rich, creamy sauce generally used to embellish vegetables, fish, and egg dishes.

HORS d' OEUVRE: Small savory appetizers served before a meal.

HOT PEPPER: Hot fresh or dried red chilis, vinegar and salt e.g., Tabasco sauce.

INFUSE: To steep an aromatic ingredient in hot liquid until the flavor has been extracted and absorbed in the liquids. Teas are infusions.

JUS: The name given to cooking juice produced during cooking. It is used to describe brown stock prepared from various kinds of meats.

LIAISON: A binding and thickening for soups and sauces. The process of thickening a sauce or soup, which includes all roux's (starch, water, slurries, beurre manière, panada and egg yolks), with or without cream.

LIQUERS: A strong sweet alcoholic spirit usually drunk after a meal. An alcoholic beverage made from a distilled spirit that has been flavored with fruit, cream, herbs, spices, flowers, or nuts bottled with added sugar, or other sweeteners. Liquers are sweet and often syrup in consistency with 15-30% alcohol by volume (ABV). In the USA it is called cordials and schnapps.

LIQUOR: Alcoholic drinks especially distilled spirits. Liquor is the name for liqueur in the USA and Canada. Liquor has 55% alcohol by volume.

MACERATE: Soaking fruits or vegetables in wine, liquor, or syrup so that they may absorb these flavors.

MARINADE: A mixture based on vinegar, lemon juice, butter milk, or yogurt with onions and other vegetables, spices, and herbs. Meat or fish is steeped in the mixture for several hours to make it tender and enhance its flavor. Marinades can also be used for dressing salads or for marinating meat that is already tender.

MARINATING: Steeping meat or fish in a liquid containing salt, wine, vinegar, lemon juice, or milk and flavorings such as herbs and spices.

MINCE: To cut food into very tiny pieces. Minced food is cut into smaller, finer pieces than diced food.

MIREPOIX: Finely diced vegetables, often with the addition of bacon and herbs, fried in butter and used as a basis for sauces.

MUFFINS: Round, flat rolls made with yeast dough and baked. In America, muffins are sweet rolls, using baking powder as a raising agent, made in special muffin pans.

PANFRY: To cook in a small amount of fat.

PARBOIL: To boil food briefly in water, cooking it partially.

PEEL: To remove the peels from vegetables and fruits.

PEPPER: The most common of all savory spices. It is best when freshly groundd or coarsely cracked or crushed from whole peppercorns.

PEPPERCORNS: The berries from vine used whole or ground as a spice.

PIE: A sweet or savory dish baked in a pastry shell with a pastry top. It is made in a pie tin (pan) with slantd-edge 5cm high. The lid of dough should have a small opening in the middle so that the steam can escape, preventing the pie crust from swelling up.

PUFF PASTRY: A light, flaky pastry made by repeatedly layering dough and butter, or another solid fat, to form thin dough that puffs in the oven.

PUREE: To grind or mash vegetables, fruits, meats, etc. until completely smooth, reduced to a pulp then cooked and sieved. A type of soup which is largely thickened by its own ingredients passed through a sieve. A purée is cooked food usually vegetables or legumes, that have been ground, pressed, blended, or sieved to the consistency of a soft creamy paste or thick liquid.

QUICK BREAD: Bread that is quick to make because it doesn't require kneading or rising time. The leavener is baking powder or baking soda. Biscuits, muffins, popover, and a wide variety of sweet and savory loaf breads are quick breads.

QUICHE: A dish that consists of a pastry shell filled with savory custard made of eggs, cream, seasonings, and various other ingredients such as onions, mushrooms, ham, shellfish, or herbs. The most common is Quiche Lorraine.

RAGOUT: A thick, rich, well-seasoned stew of meat, poultry or fish that can be made with or without vegetables.

RAMEKIN OR COCOTTE: A small, round, ovenproof China, or earthenware dish in which individual portions are cooked and served. They are about 8cm - 9cm in diameter and they can be used for both sweet and savory dishes, either baked or chilled.

RATATOUILLE: A popular dish from the French region of Provence that combines eggplant, tomatoes, onions, bell peppers, zucchini, garlic, and herbs, all simmered in olive oil. The vegetables can vary according to the cook. They can be cooked together or separately and then combined and heated briefly. Ratatouille can be served hot, cold, or at room temperature, either as a side dish or as an appetizer with bread or crackers.

RED ONIONS (SPANISH ONIONS): Are medium to large onions that have purplish red skins and red-tinged white flesh with a mild sweet flavor.

RED WINE VINEGARS: Made from red wine, is more robust and pungent than vinegar made from white wine.

REDUCE: To boil liquid (usually stock, wine, or a sauce mixture) rapidly until the volume is reduced by evaporation, thereby thickening the consistency, and intensifying the flavor. Such a mixture is sometimes referred to as a reduction.

ROUX: A mixture of flour and fat after being slowly cooked over low heat. It is used to thicken mixtures such as soups and sauces. There are three classic roux - white, blond, and brown. The color and flavor is determined by the length of time the mixture is cooked.

SAUTE: To fry quickly in a little hot fat. Cooked or browned in a pan containing a small quantity of butter, oil, or other fat.

SCALD: To heat a liquid to just under boiling point e.g., milk. To pour boiling water over tomatoes in order to remove skin.

SEA SALT: A result of evaporation of sea water. It comes in fine grains or large crystals.

SELF-RISING FLOUR: Generally all-purpose flour, to which a leavening agent has been added, in the form of baking powder and salt. The type of flour used in many packed mixes such as cake batters. 1 cup of self-rising flour equal to 1 cup all-purpose flour, plus 1½ teaspoons baking powder and 1 teaspoon salt.

SHALLOT: The member of the onion family, with papery brown skin, purple-tinged white flesh and a flavor resembling a cross between sweet onion and garlic.

SHERBET: A frozen dessert made from unsweetened fruit juice and water, sherbet is lighter than ice cream, but richer than ice cream and sorbet.

SHORT BREAD: A rich crumbly cookie made of butter, flour, and sugar.

SIMMER: To cook slowly just below boiling point while bubbling gently.

SORBET: French name for "sherbet" is a smooth soft, frozen dish made of puréed fruit or fruit juice and sugar. It doesn't contain milk, sometimes flavored with wine or liqueur. It is served as a palate cleanser between courses or as dessert. Also referred to as ice or granita, but these have a grainier texture than sorbet

SOUFFLE: Particularly light, aerated dish made with beaten egg white which maybe sweet or savory.

SOUR CREAM: A commercial dairy product made from pasteurized sweet cream, has tangy flavor and thick consistency used to enrich savory and sweet recipes or as a topping. Like buttermilk its extra acidity boosts the leavening action of baking soda.

STRAINING: Filter solid matter from liquids or draining liquids from raw or cooked foods.

SUPREME: Breast of chicken or game. The breast refers to the best part of a bird which is always prepared with the greatest care.

TARTLET: Small tart made from short crust or puff pastry with a sweet or savoring filling.

THICKENING: The addition of a substance to a sauce or soup to thicken it. Flour, roux, egg yolk or cream can be used to thicken soups. Egg yolk or cream can be stirred into the liquid to make an emulsion.

TIMBALE: A mold lined with pastry, blind-baked and filled with meat, fish, or other ingredients in a sauce, baked in the oven or cooked in a bain-marie.

TURNING: Forming vegetables and potatoes into decorative shapes such as balls, ovals, spirals.

WORCESTERSHIRE SAUCE: A traditional English seasoning or condiment is an intensely flavorful blend of many ingredients, including molasses, soy sauce, garlic, onion, and anchovies. Used as a marinade ingredient or a table sauce.

WOK: A large bowl-shaped Chinese pen used for frying food quickly in hot oil.

YOGURT: Milk fermented by bacterial cultures that impart a mildly acidic flavor and custard-like texture. Plain yogurt refers to the unflavored product.

ZUCCHINI: Slender, tuber-shaped summer squash have edible green, yellow or green-and-cream skin and pale, tender flesh.

ZEST: The thin outer rind of oranges or lemons, used for its flavor and fragrance. It is the thin, brightly colored outermost layer of the peel of a citrus fruit, containing most of the peel's aromatic essential oils. It provides lively flavor to both sweet and savory dishes.

CULINARY AND MEDICINAL HERBS USED IN CAMEROON CUISINE

Herbs are parts of leafy green plants such as basil, oregano, thyme, rosemary, parsley, and mint, used for flavoring food, or as a garnish. Herbs can be aromatic, such as mentha and inoffensive such as parsley, thyme, chervil, and bay leaves. An herb can also be defined as any "seed-bearing annual, biennial, or perennial plant that does not develop persistent woody tissue but dies down at the end of a growing season." {Unlike a tree for instance} or "a plant or plant part valued for its medicinal, savory or aromatic qualities"

A spice is any plant product except the leaves used primarily for seasoning food. It is usually dried and may be a seed, fruit, root, bark berry, bud, twigs, or vegetable substance, such as cinnamon, ginger, chili, cloves, and mustard seed. Spices are rich in iron, trace metals, and potassium. They can have a violent action which can irritate the digestive tract, such as hot pepper, ginger, and white pepper.

Condiments are seasonings, such as mustard, ketchup, salt, spices, vinegar, or relish added to food at the table to give a special flavor or complement. Spices are rich in iron, trace metals, and potassium. Spices can have a violent action which can irritate the digestive tract, such as hot pepper, ginger, and white pepper.

Cameroon, like all other African countries uses a lot of spices and herbs in their cooking. In Cameroon both imported and local indigenous spices are used. These spices come from the Equatorial rain forests of the country. The leaves, barks, roots, and stems are used. Most often the spices are dried, sold whole, or ground into powder. Most of the spices belong to the pepper family and have many medicinal values. The green herbs of basil, celery, and parsley are usually called green spices and are grown by local farmers which are used in a majority of dishes. Imported spices are found in supermarkets in the major cities of the country.

THE ROLE OF CULINARY SPICES

1. Flavoring agent such as cardamom (odzom).
2. Preservations such as garlic, turmeric, and fenugreek powder.
3. Souring agent such as tamarind.
4. Thickening agent such as poppy seeds, ginger, and garlic paste.
5. Medicinal agents such as coriander seeds and cumin seeds, which aids in digestion, garlic and onions help reduce blood sugar and cholesterol levels.
6. Stimulants such as in the digestive glands and the appetite.
7. Imparts variety in foods because different spices give different colors, flavors, and taste to food.
8. They give pungency such as chilies and ginger.

AFRICAN AND CAMEROONIAN CULINARY SPICES

SN	ENGLISH NAME	FRENCH NAME	BOTANICAL NAME	COMMON NAME
1.	African Nutmeg	Faux noix de muscade	Monodora myristica	Medjock and Meridak (Bamileke), Calabash nutmeg Pébè (Cameroon), Jamaica nutmeg, ehuru, ehiri, ariwo, airama, African orchid nutmeg, muscadier de calabash, Lubushi, awarewa, Fake nutmeg, Nding and Hikoma (Bassa)
2.	Aridan		Tetrapleura tetraptera	Eseke-seke (Cameroon) Preseke (Ghana) 4 sides Esésè
3.	Bastered melegueta	Mariguette suerée	a) Aframomium danielli Aframomium Citrantum	Mbongo (Cameroon) Bongolo Tchouoko Atare, ósè, oji Indokoja mokpe (Bakweri)
4.	Grains of paradise Seed of Heaven		b) Aframomium melegueta c) Afromomium sp uganda	Mbongo (Cameroon) Alligator pepper (Cameroon) Hepper pepper, Guinea grains, Fom wisa, atariko, ataecko, Meleguetta pepper, atare (Nigeria), ata-ire Seed of Eding
5.	Country onion	Oignon sauvage	Afrostyrax lepidophyllus	Ngakanga Bush onion (Cameroon) Lumtom Foulon (Ngemba) L'olum
6.	African black pepper	Poivre noir poivre sauvage	Piper nigrum	Pepe Piper

7.	Ethiopian pepper	Poivre d'Ethiopie	Xylopia aethiopica	Kieng (Ngemba) Bikwi (Bamileke) Grains of selim, uda, Kimba pepper, African pepper Moor pepper Negro pepper Kani pepper Senegal pepper Whentia pepper (Ghana) Guinea pepper Djar (Senegal) Kili pepper
8.	Seed of African locust beans paste	Grain de caroube	Parkia biglobosa	Dawa-dawa (Ghana) Iru, néré, ugba Carob, dadawa
9.	Sichuan pepper	Bouche béante	a) Fogara xanthoxyloide b) Fogara leprie c) Fogara tessman	Chinese coriander Ngachu'u (Bamileke) Natchou (Bamileke) Wild lime, Colima, una degato Corriosa
10.	Carterpillar plant		Hypodaphnis zenkeri	Nkouppo (Bamileke) Prickly caterpillar Prickly scorpion tail Bunte Davida
			Pentadiplandra	Oubli
11.	Globe thistles		Echinops giganteus	Tchanmgne, kessa, Ayilagwen, kahgoh Tsegum Soapte
12.	African Davida	a) Fruit de l'arbe à l'ail b) Ecorce rouge.	Scorodophloeus zenkeri	Hyiomi, hiomi Omi plat, Akob (Ngemba) Kanda stick
13.	Seed of heaven		Afromomium sp Uganda	Atzoh (Ngemba) Ndong (Cameroon) Wild cardamom Guinea pepper African pepper
14.	Striped African pepper	Poivre de sédhiou	Xylopia parviflora	Nkey

15.	West African pepper		Piper guineese	Soppe (Ngemba) Jowe (Cameroon) Ashanti pepper Benin pepper False cubeb Guinea cubeb Uziza pepper Kale, masoro, Kukauabe, sasema Soro wisa
16.	African mango	Grains de mangues sauvages	Irvingia gabonensis	Ndotuah (East) Bush mango seed (Cameroon) Wild mango (Cameroo) Dika nuts (Nigeria) Ogwono (Nigeria) Njaka Ndo'o (East Region) Manguis (Sanbage) Mfiang Ndog (Beti, Betsi, Fang) Chocolate (Gabon) Mango sauce.
17.	African wood-oil nut	Graine de ricin	Ricinodendron heudelottü Ricinodendron africanum	Essessang, djansang, Essang, ezezang, njasang, Njangsa, njangsanga (Cameroon) Munguella (Angola) Bofeko (RDC) Wama (Ghana) Okhuen (Nigeria) Kishongo (Uganda) Akpi (Cote d'Ivoire) Ricin grains Omega – 3 seeds
18.	African bread fruit		Treculia Africana	Phembi, ukwa
19.	Pumpkin seed	Grains de courge	Cucubita pepo seeds	Pepita (Spanish) Green egusi (Cameroon) Ngeehniboh (Ngemba)

20.	White seed melon Gourd seeds	Pistache	Cucumeropsis mannii Mann's cucumeropsis	Ngeeh (Ngemba) Ngondo (Douala) Nnam Ngon (Yaounde) Egusi (Yoruba) Agushi (Hausa) Nju (West Region) Country egusi (Cameroon) Egusi – itoo Melon seeds, Ibo egusi The real egusi Ibo egusi Calabash egusi.
21.	Groundnuts	Arachides	Arachis hypogaea	Ngon (Yaounde) Munzhu (Ngemba) Peanut.
22.	Bambara groundnuts		Voandzeia subterranean	Ndzou (Ngemba, Cameroon) Congo groundnuts Congo goobar Madasgascar groundnuts Earth pea Njugo bean (South African) Voandzou nzama (Malawi) Inolhlubu Underground bean.
23.	Soya beans	Le soja	Glycine max	Soybean (North American) Soya bean (Europe)
24.	Bird's eye pepper	Petit piment	Capsicum frutescen Capsicum annum	Chili pepper Jelapeno, habeno, serano, Thai pepper, pili-pili
25.	Prickly ash		Fogara Leprieulli Zanthoxylum heitzii Fogara heitzii	Melan
26.	Alligator pepper		Fogara tessmanoii	Mbongo Uzazi
27. 28.	White ginger	Gingembre Blanc La racine Hypodaphais zenkeri	Mondio whitei	Mondio, mondo, la racine, tonic root, mundodo, lintse, nkang bongo (chalk)
29.			Pentadepladra brazzeana	Ghomala'a (Baham), Lokele, Osimi Dambeno (Central African Rep.) Busini (RDC)

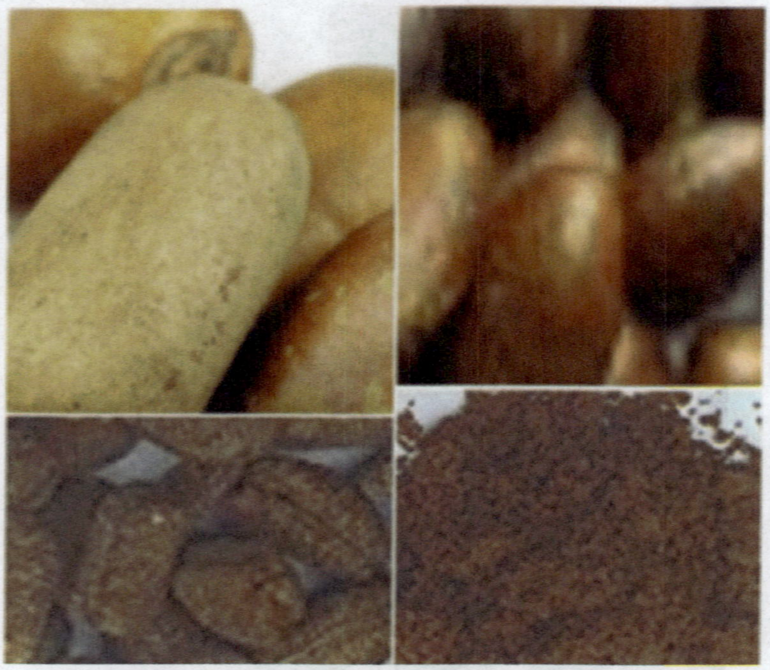

Monodora myristica (African nutmeg, Calabash nutmeg, Pe'be', Medjock)

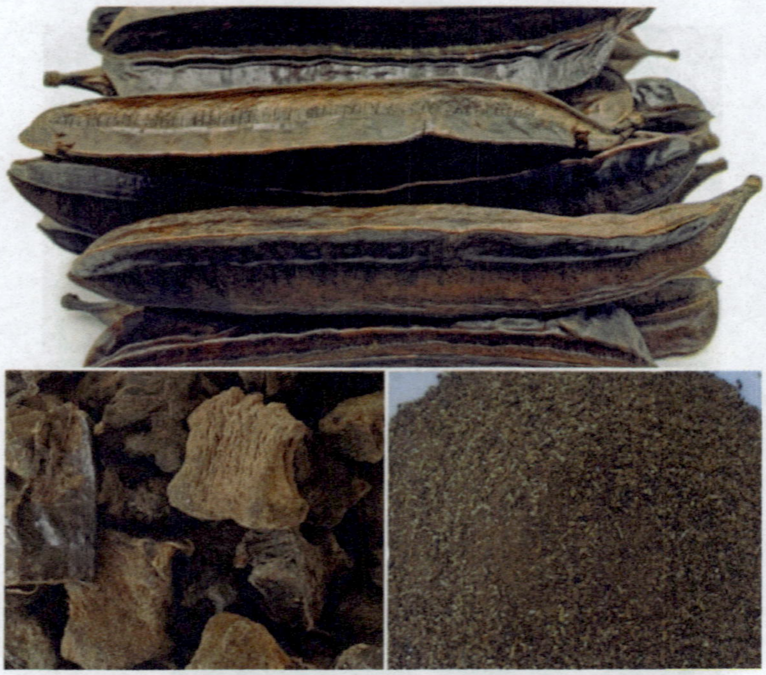

Tetrapleura tetraptera (Eseke-seke, 4 sides, preseke)

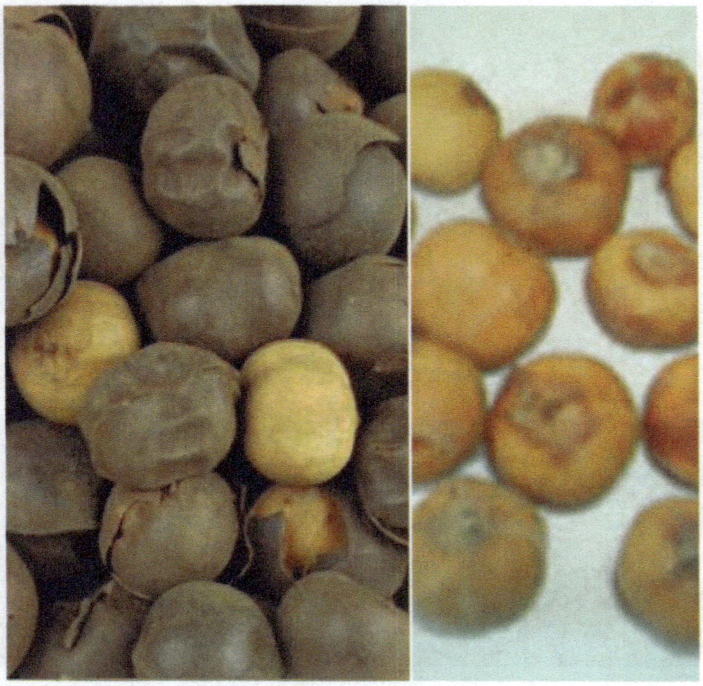

Afrostyrax lepidophyllus (Bush onion, Foulom, Ngakanga)

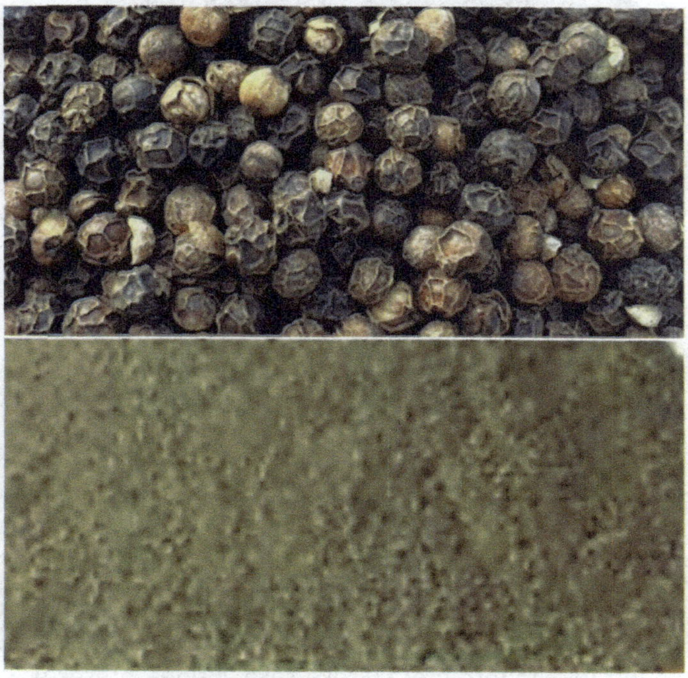

Piper nigrum (African black pepper, pepe, poivre savage, piper)

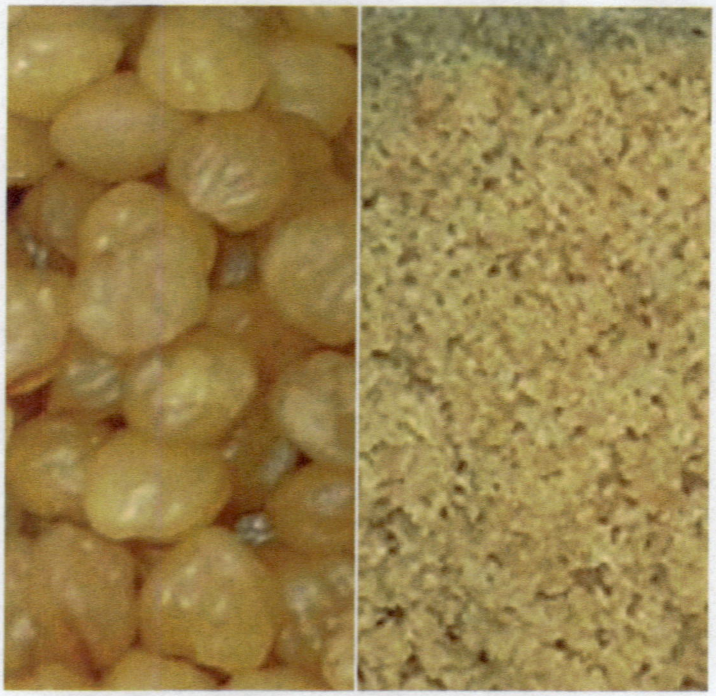

Recinodendron heudelottu (Njangsa, Akpi, omega-3 seeds, essessang. Wama, kishongo)

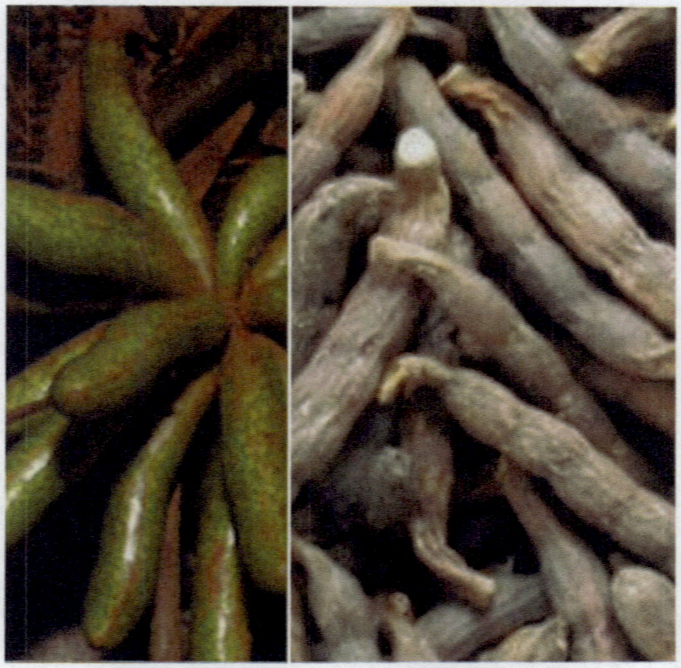

Xlopia aethiopica (Bikwi, African pepper,kieng, Ethiopian pepper, grains of selim)

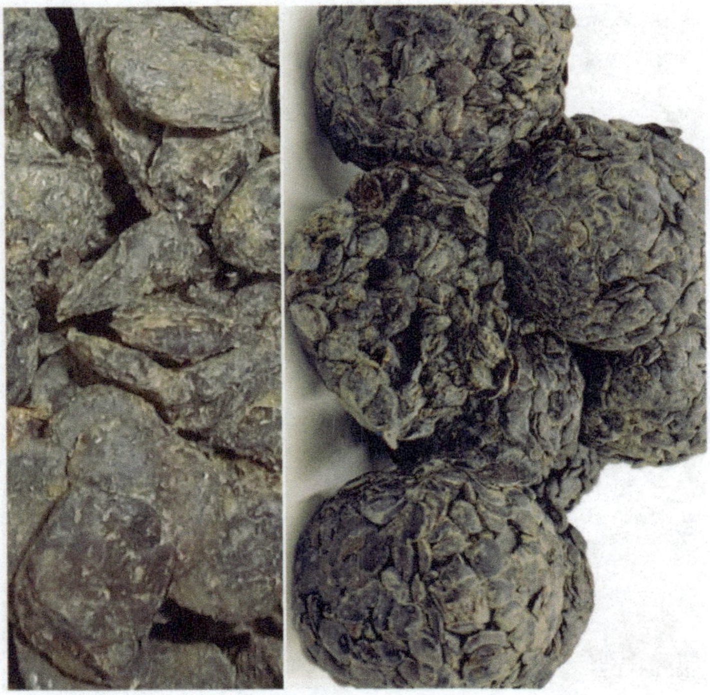

Parkia biglobosa (Dawa-dawa, carob, dadawa, Iru)

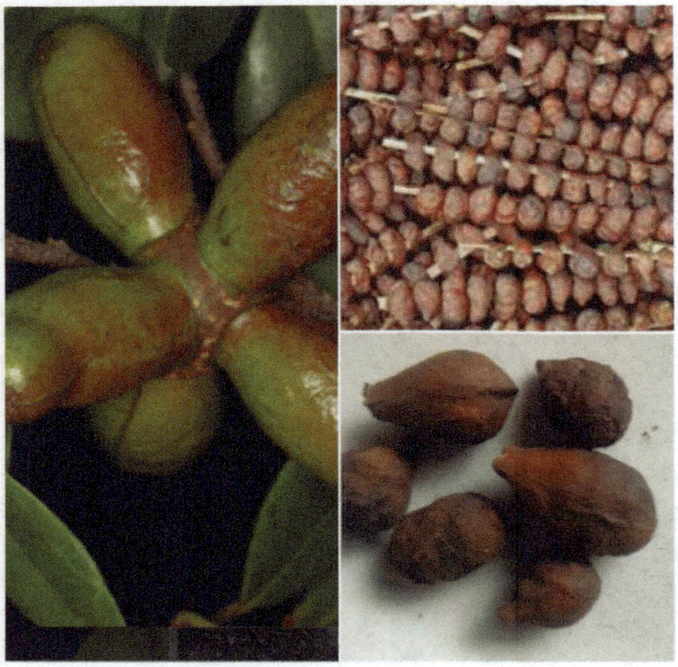

Xylopia parviflora (Striped African pepper, poivre de Se'dhiou)

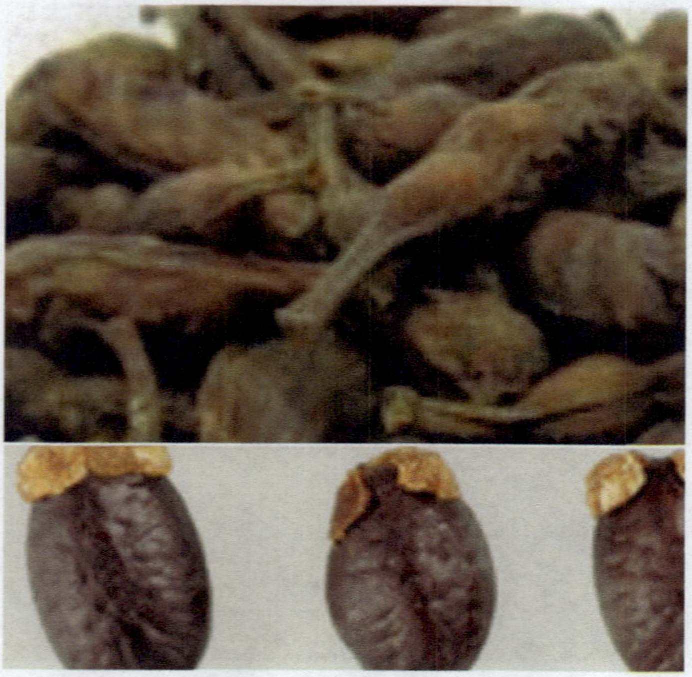

Xylopia aromatic (kieng)

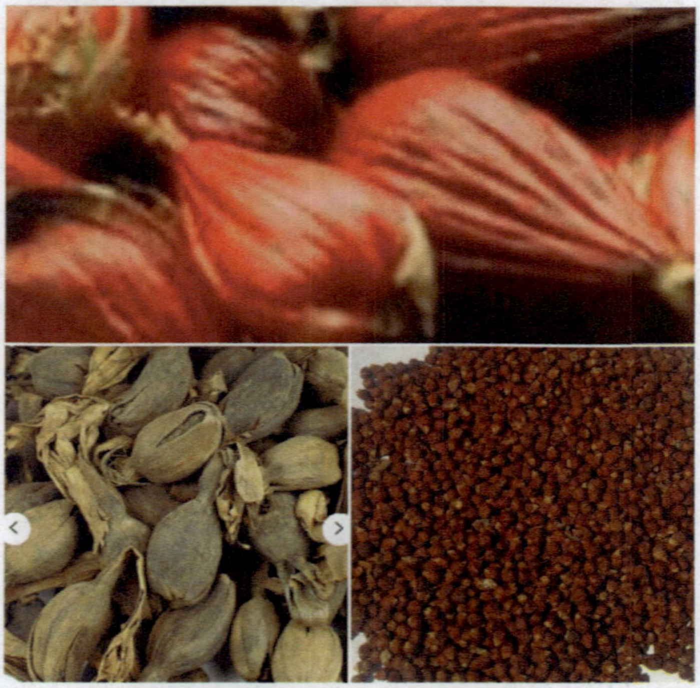

Afromomium melegueta (mbongo)

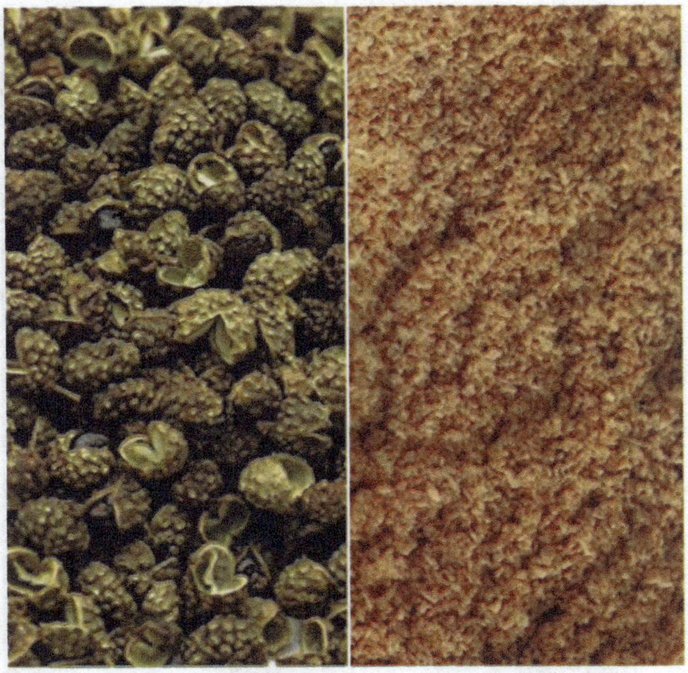

Fagara xanthoxyloides (Sichuan pepper, Chinese coriander, Ngachu'u, natchou?

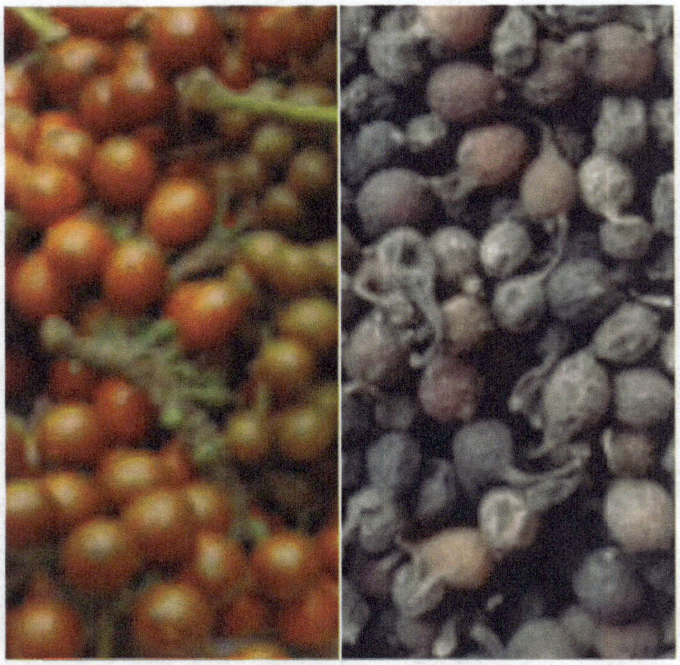

Piper guineese (West African pepper, sopp, jowe, uziza pepper, Ashanti pepper

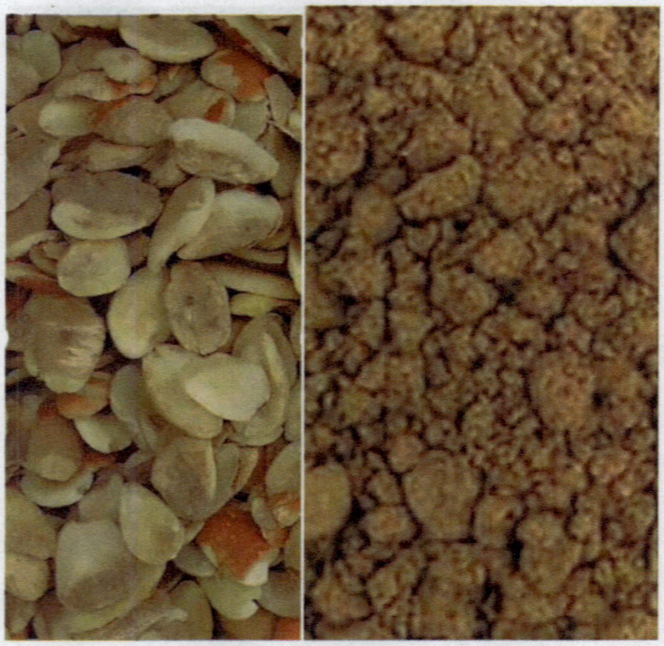

Irvingia gabonensis (Ndotuah, bush mango, ogwono, ndo'o, wild mango)

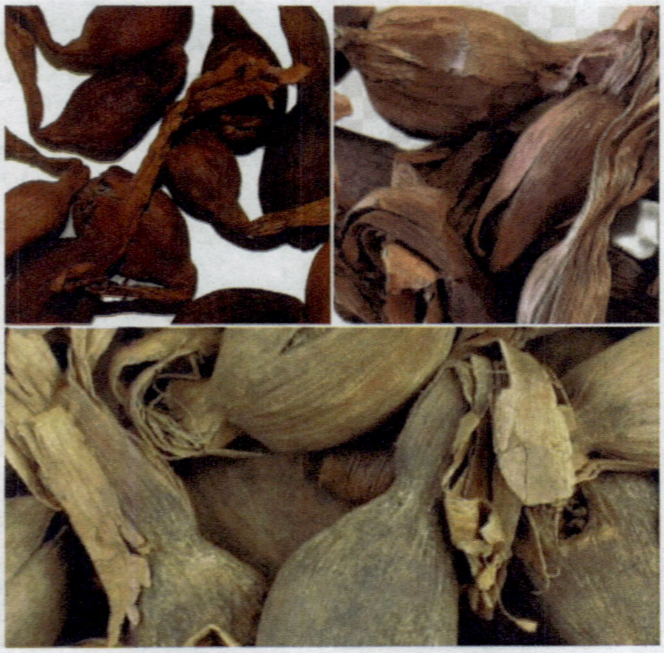

Afromomium danielli and Afromomium melegueta (Mbongo, bongolo, tchouoko)

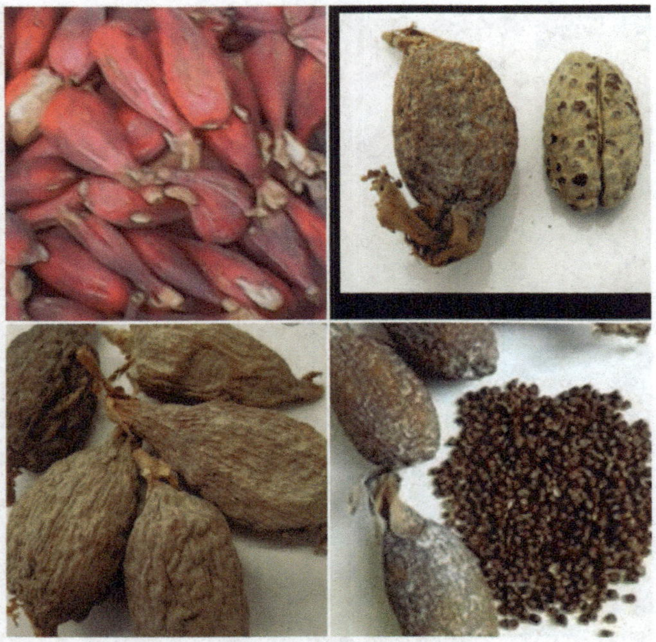

Afromomium citrantum (Atare, mokpe, alligator pepper)

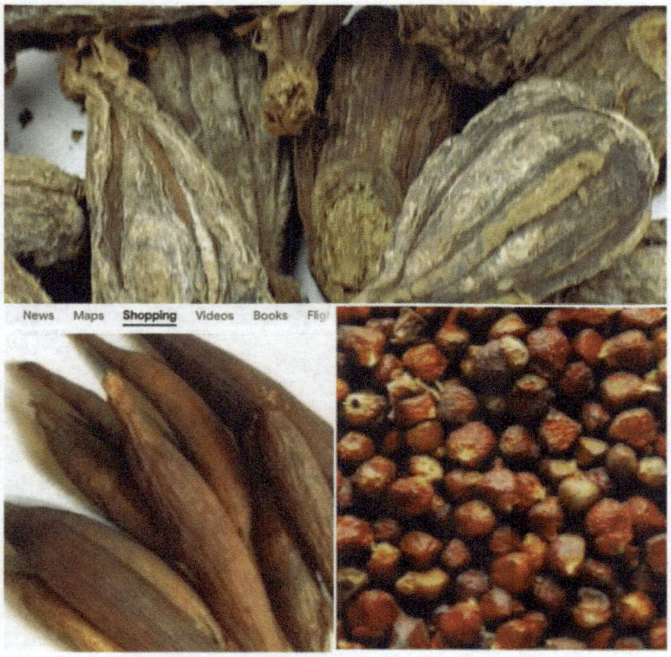

Tchobi, ndong, grains of paradise

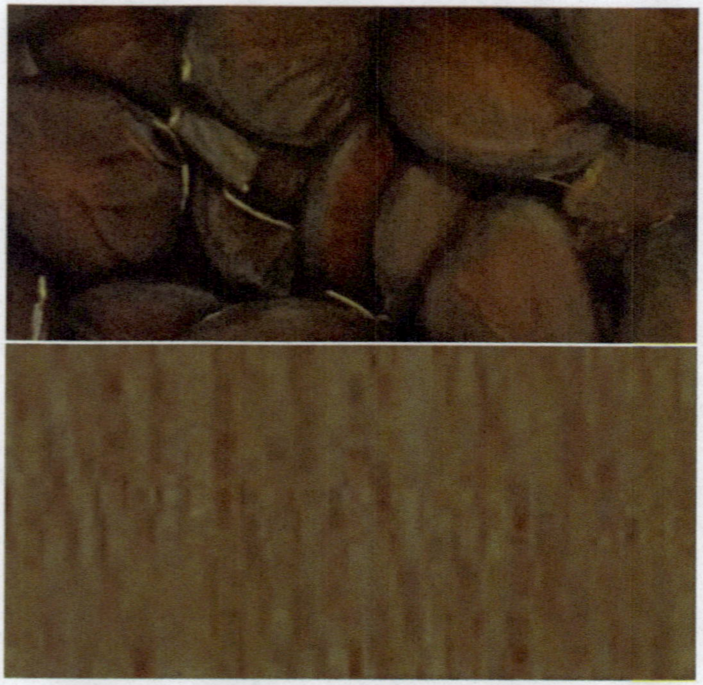

Scorodophloeus zenkeri (lem, lom, Doum, hiomi, Olam,bobinbi, olom, button). Kanda stick, akob.

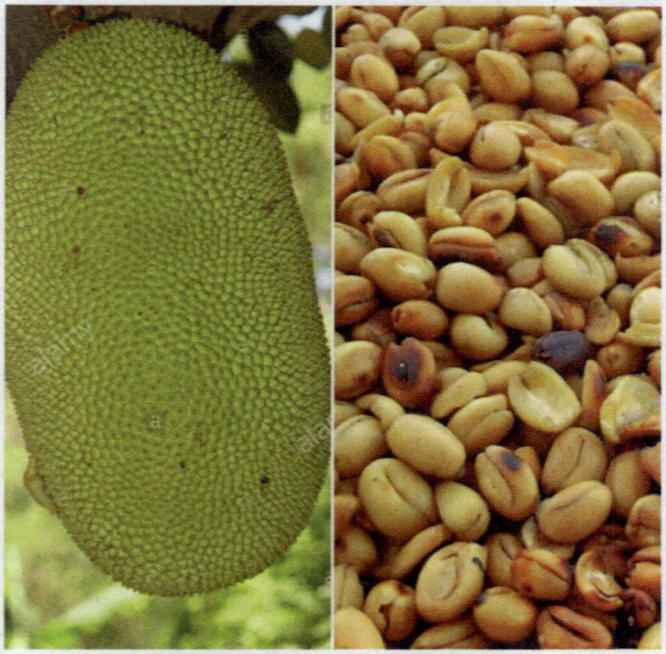

Treculia africana (phembi, ukwa seeds)

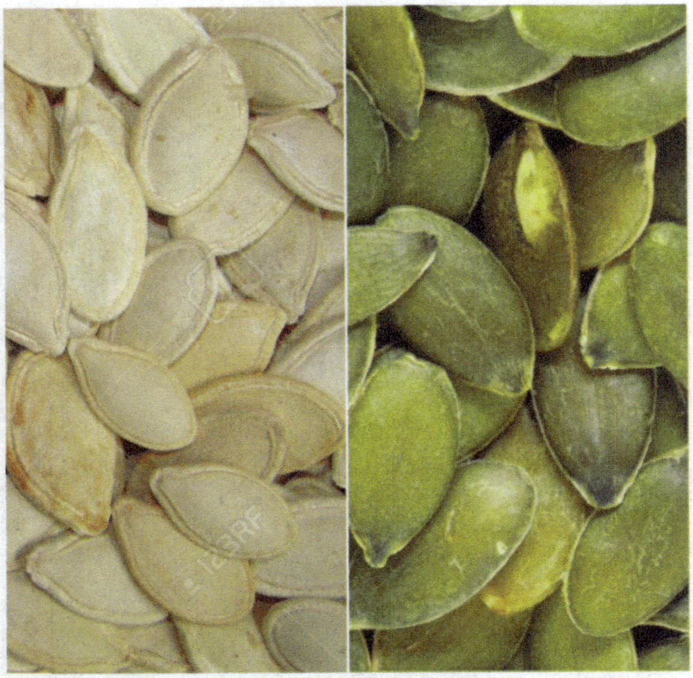

Cucubita pepo seed (green egusi, pumpkin seeds, melon seeds.)

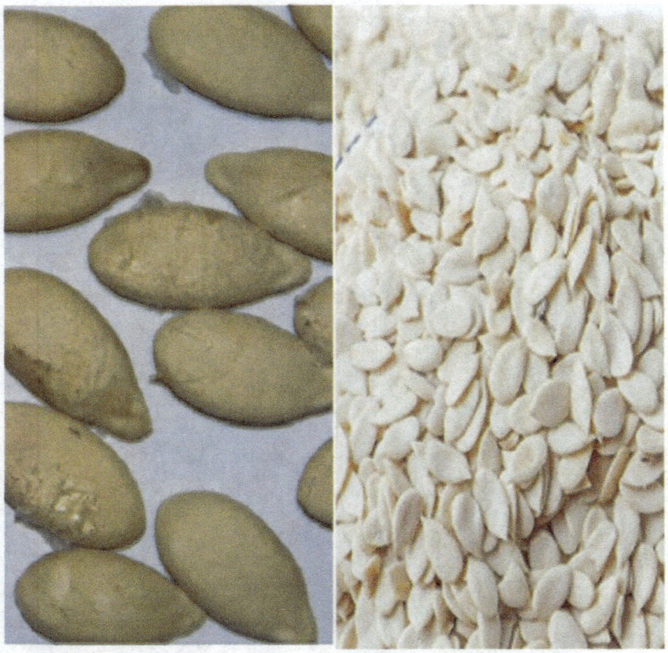

Cucumeropsis mannii (ngondo, ngeeh, nnam ngon, white egusi, Ibo egusi, meon seeds)

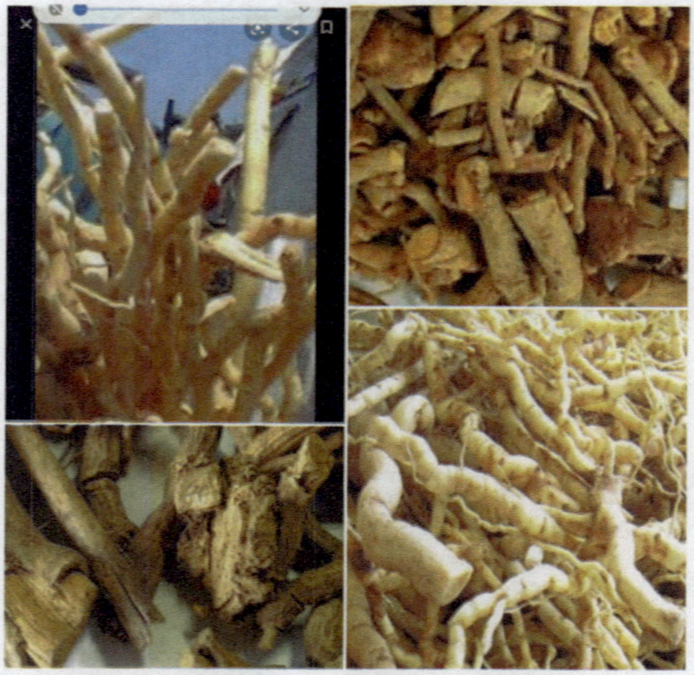

Mondio whiteii (African Mulino, mondo, nkang bongo)

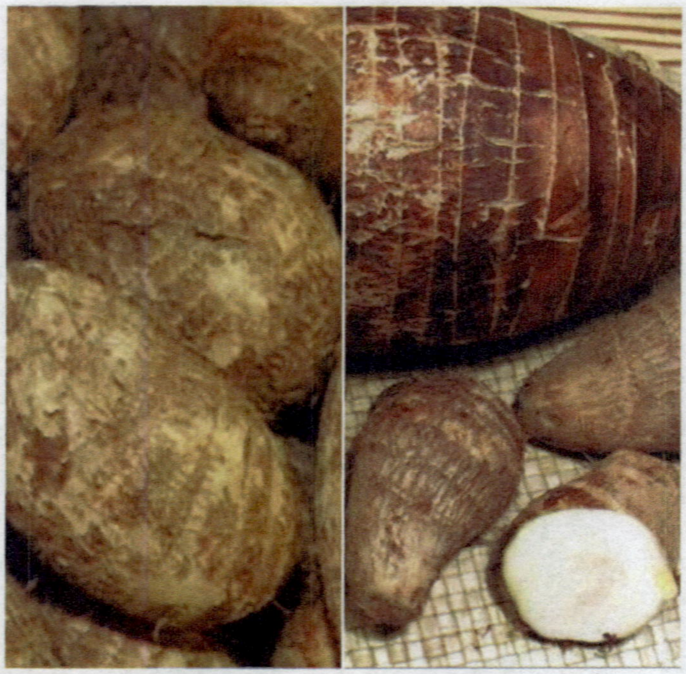

Colocasia esculenta (Ibo cocoyams, Taro, Japanese Taro)

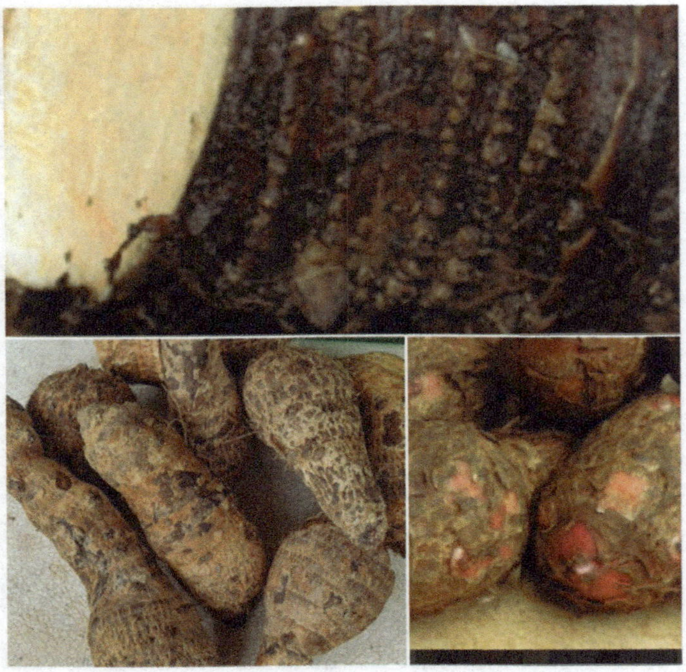

Xanthosoma sagittifolium (macabo, malanga)

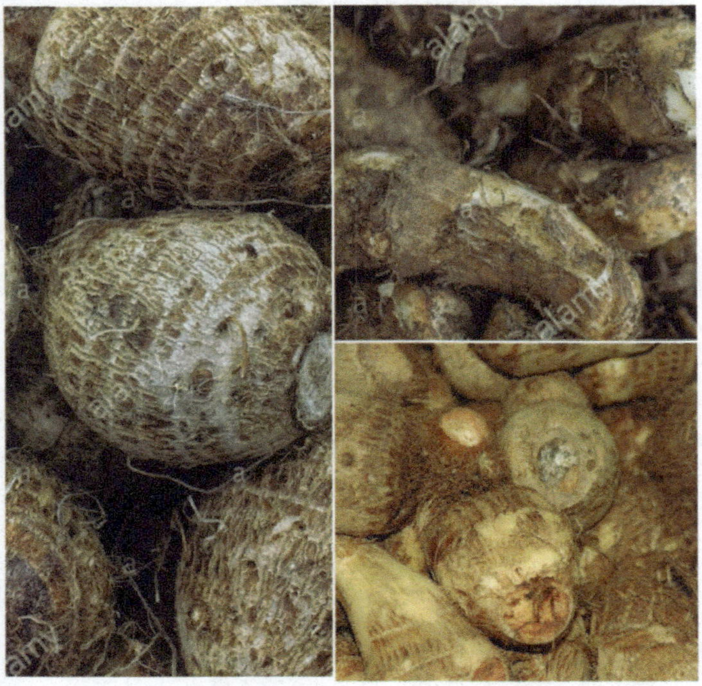

Colocasia antiquorium (country cocoyams, nku-uh)

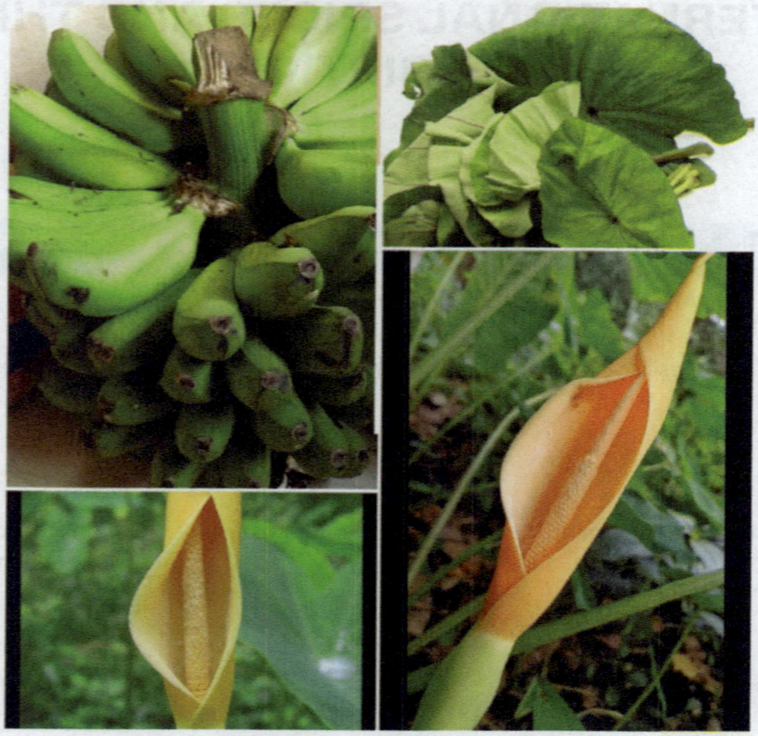

Achu banana, Taro leaves, Taro flowers or blossom.

INTERNATIONAL SPICES AND THEIR DESCRIPTIONS

	English name	French name	Botanical name	Common name
1.	Anis	Anis vert	Pimpinella anisum	Suva Aniseed
2	Basil	Basilic	Ocimum basilicum	"king of herbs" St. St Joseph's – Wort Great Basil Royal Basil Sweet Basil
	African Basil	Basilic à petit Feuille	Ocimum gratissimum	Efinrin (Yoruba) L'Ossim Nnam (Yde) Clove Basil Anigbe Kotmargin
	Wild basil	Basilic sauvage		Massep (Beti) Massip Masepo (Tropical Basil)
3	Bay leaf	Feuille de laurier	Laurus nobilis	Laurel
4	Celery	Celeri	Apium graveolens	Celeriac (root celery)
5	Chives	Ciboulette civet	Allium graveolens	Celeriac (root celery)
6	Cloves	Clou de girofle	Allium schoenoprasum	
7	Coriander	Coriandre	Coriandrum sativum	Cilantro (America) Chinese parsley Dhania (India)
8	Cumin	Cumin	Cuminum cyminum	
9	Garlic	Ail	Allium sativum	
10	Ginger	Gingembre	Zingiber officinate	Gyin (Burma) Halia (Malaysia)
	Ginger leaves	Feuille d'Odzom	Zingiber officinale.	Feuille d'odzom Munjuweli
11	Leeks	Poireau	Allium am peloprasum L.	Spring onions
12	Mentha	Menthe	Lamiaceae	Mint
13	Nutmeg	Muscade Noir de muscade	Myristica fragrans	Pala (Indonesia) Noce Moscala **(Italian)**
14	Onions	Oignon	Allium cepa	

15	Oregano	Origan	Oreganum vulgare	Wild marjoram Mexican thyme Mexican mint
16	Parsley	Persil Cumin	Petrolselinum Crispum	Commun parsley Garden parsley
17	Rosemary	Rosmarin	Rosmarinus Officinalis	Anthos
18	Sesame seeds	Graines de sesame	Sesamum Indicum	
19	Spear mint	La menthe en epi	Mentha spicata	Mentha crepue Menthe douce
20	Turmeric	Curcuma	Curcuma longa	Yellow ginger
21	Thyme	Thym	Thymus vulgaris	Common thyme German thyme
22	Shallot	Echalotte		Scallion
23	savory	Sariette		
24	Dill	Aneth		
25	Cinnamon		Cinnamon verum	
26	Fenugreek		Trigonella foenum-graecum	Leeks

"I give you every seed-bearing plant on the face of the whole earth and any tree that has fruit with seed in it. This will be yours for food." (Gen. 1:2 NIV).

The Bible mentions 128 plants that were part of the everyday life of ancient Israel, and of its Mediterranean neighbors. The bible often mentions herbs, they were highly valued in biblical times. Natural herbs offer medicines for inducing healing, preserving health, and improving our quality of life.

Dr. Jordan S. Rubin, a doctor of naturopathic medicine and a certified nutritional consultant, in his book *"The Maker's Diet,"* has listed twenty-one of the top biblical herbs as follows: Aloes, Black cumin (Nigella sativa), Black mustard (brassica nigra), Cinnamon (Cinnamomum verum), Coriander(Coriandrum sativum), Cumin(Cuminum cyminum), Dandelion(Taraxacum officinale), Dill(Anethum graveolens), Henna (Lawsonia inermis), Frankincense (Trigonella foenum-graecum), Frankincense (Boswellia sacra), Garlic (Allium sativum), Hyssop (Hyssopus officinalis or Origanum syriacum), Juniper (Juniperus oxycedrus), Milk Thistle (Silybum marianum), Mint or horse mint (Mentha longifolia),

Myrrh (Cistus inamus or Commiphora erythraea), Nettle or Stinging nettles (Urtica dioica), Saffron (Crocus sativus), herbs Spikenard (Nardostachys grandiflora or jatamansi), and Turmeric (Curcuma longa).

Many of these herbs are used as seasonings, some are edible in salads or soups, and some can be used to make teas. Ten of these herbs (cumin, cinnamon, coriander, dill, fenugreek, garlic, oregano(hyssop), mint, saffron, turmeric) are found in this book and are used as spices. Dandelion is one of the bitter herbs eaten at the Passover.

DESCRIPTION OF SOME SPICES AND HERBS

Anise: It is a spice whose flavor is reminiscent of licorice, usually bought whole, crushed, or ground. It is of the parsley family. It is used in cookies, cakes, liqueurs, and savory dishes such as seasoning and marinades of fish. Other names are aniseed and Suva. Two-star anise is called badiane.

Basil: It is the "king" of all fresh herbs used in the kitchen. It is a member of the mint family that has a pungent smell. It can be used both fresh and dry and in a variety of dishes such as salads. Basil is of many varieties such as Royal Basil, African Basil, and wild basil. It has many medicinal values. African Basil is kotmargin, wild basil is massepu.

Bay leaf: It is a leaf similar to the Eucalyptus leaf, but from the bay laurel. It can be used whole, halved, or ground. It lends a slightly bitter, pungent seasoning to soups, stews, and stocks. It is also known as laurel. It is one of the primary ingredients of a bouquet garni.

Black Pepper: This is the most widely traded spice in the world. It is dried in its peelings.

Cinnamon (Cinnamomum verum): It was part of the holy anointing oil used to anoint the priests and vessels in the Tabernacle of Moses. (EX. 30:22-25). It was also mentioned in setting the stage for romance (Prov. 7:17-18). It calms the stomach and may even prevent ulcers. Cinnamon contains benzaldehyde, and anti-tumor agent, antiseptic properties that kill bacteria- causing tooth decay and disease-causing fungi and viruses. It may prevent urinary tract infection (UTI) and infestation of candida. Cinnamon reduces the amount of insulin necessary for glucose metabolism in Type 11 diabetes. 1/8 teaspoon of this herb triples insulin efficiency.

Coriander (Coriandrum sativum): (Cilantro) Also known as Chinese parsley. It resembles and is often used as parsley. The dried seeds of this aromatic plant are called coriander. This spice is used whole or ground. It is used traditionally as a remedy for acid digestion, neuralgia, rheumatism, and toothaches. Research shows that it can aid in elimination of harmful metals from the body, including mercury, lead and cadmium. Coriander contains 21 natural chemicals possessing antibacterial properties that help control body odor. It's essential oil treats indigestion and excess gas.

Cloves: It is brown, hard, dried flower buds of an aromatic evergreen tree. It is an intensely spicy aromatic, bitter, and woody taste. When they are ground, they are used in cakes and soups, but when they are whole, they add flavor to mulled wines, cider as well as cooking whole hams. Cloves are also used in marinades, red cabbage, and braised dishes.

Cumin (Cuminum cyminum): Originally it is an Indian spice with an earthly flavor. It is a fundamental ingredient of curry powder and curry pastes used for braised dishes such as beef, lamb or kid, ground or whole. It is also known as Comino or Cuminum cyminum. It has antioxidant properties and was used in the biblical times as a medicine and appetite stimulant. It is a remedy for arrhythmia (abnormal heartbeat) asthma, dermatitis, and impotence. The aromatic oil of this aromatic seed was used as a disinfectant, because it is bactericidal and larvicidal and it possesses anesthetic properties. Research shows that the spice contains three pain-relieving compounds and seven anti-inflammatory properties.

Curry powder: A spice mixture of many spices of almost thirty of them common to India. It usually consists of coriander, turmeric, fenugreek, cumin, ginger, garlic, clove, cayenne, and other chilies, caraway, and all spice. It is used to add flavor to meat, fish, and poultry dishes.

Fenugreek (Trigonella foenum-graecum): This herb maybe what the Bible calls "leeks". It contains five compounds that appear to help diabetics' lower blood pressure.

Ginger: It is the thick gnarled root of a tropical plant used for its spicy aromatic rhizome. It has a sharp fruit aroma and adds an exotic touch to both savory dishes as curries, marinades, rice, tea, and sweet dishes. It is also known as green or root ginger.

Hyssop (Hyssopus officinalis or Origanum syriacum): It is also called Marjoram. A spice, a tonic, and a digestive aid, hyssop was the "Bible's brush of salvation" used for spreading the blood of lambs on door posts to spare the Israelites from the angel of death in Egypt. It was also use in purification ceremonies to cleanse those who came into contact with lepers and corpses. Hyssops stops bleeding (as an astringent) and effectively masks odors. It was used traditionally as a remedy for colds, inflammation, and rheumatism. It has been used as a digestive aid.

Dill (Anethum graveolens): It is a remedy for cancer and estrogen deficiency, a digestive aid, and a remedy for excessive internal gas. Dill seed oil inhibits the growth of several bacteria that attached to the digestive tract. As a tea, it soothes the stomach and intestines and also relieves upper respiratory ailments. Its oil is strongly antibacterial that inhibits organisms such as Bacillus anthracis. Dill contains various phytochemicals that act as insecticides, enhances estrogen levels, fight infection, bacteria, and insects, acts as a uterine relaxant.

Mint or Horse mint (Mentha longifolia): Mint or "sweet-scented plants" are mentioned in two Gospels (Mt 23:23, Lk 11:42). Some species of mint are used to treat Alzheimer's disease and to flavor candies, gum, toothpaste, and liqueurs. They are used as digestive aids. Peppermint oil is antiallergenic and it is used in aromatherapy to stimulate brain activity. Mint is also used in a variety of food dishes such as soups, salads, meat dishes, and often added to potatoes and peas. It is delicious as mint tea, and the leaves are used for decoction. It is also known as mentha.

Nutmeg: It is the oval, brown, wrinkled seed of the nutmeg tree. It is used grated as a spice for both sweet and savory dishes. It is delicious in soups, stews, potato puree and cabbage.

Parsley: This is the most popular of all herbs. The roots are full of flavor and are deliciously added to soups and sauces. Parsley is rich in vitamins and minerals. There are two types of parsley, curly leaf and flat leaf which is also known as continental or Italian parsley.

Peppercorn: Dried white pepper is known as peppercorn.

Saffron (Crocus sativus): It is a flowering herb served as a condiment, sweet perfume, and coloring agent in biblical times. It was once the world's most expensive spice. 25 grams of saffron requires 4.300 flowers. Saffron was used medicinally in tinctures for treating gastric and intestinal problems and is considered antispasmodic, expectorant, sedative, and a stimulant in small doses. It is also helpful for bladder, kidney, and liver ailments.

Thyme: It is an essential part of a bouquet garni and one of the main ingredients of Herbes de Provence. Thyme gives a special touch to many dishes such as meat, fish, poultry, and vegetables.

White pepper: It is milder and more delicate in taste than, and not as sharp as, black pepper. The white peppercorn comes from the ripe fruit which is peeled before drying. This white pepper is produced in Njombe, called Njombe pepper or Steenberg's white peppercorn.

Chives: It is like shallots but smaller in size and is good for scrambled eggs.

Garlic (Allium sativum): Enhances salads, cold sauces, roast stews, braised and grilled (broiled) dishes. It is an infection fighter, and it even discourages irritating and potentially dangerous mosquitoes and ticks. It is a painkiller, stimulates the immune system, and it is helpful for treating asthma, diabetes, and high blood pressure.

Paprika: A spicy seasoning ground from a sweet variety of red pepper used to flavor ragouts, stuffing, sauces, and garnishing.

Shallots: This is an onion variety that produces clusters of bulbs. Their flavor is less intense than that of onions with a hint of garlic.

Turmeric (Curcuma longa): It is from a rhizome plant that is often dried and ground. It is used as a spice and a food color. It is sometimes called curcuma longa or yellow ginger. Turmeric has many medicinal values such as anti-inflammatory and antioxidant properties. It may be beneficial as a wound treatment, digestive aid, liver protector, and heart tonic. Its essential oil has anti-inflammatory and anti-arthritic qualities and a pain killer.

COMBINATION HERBS AND SPICES

All spice: It's a pea-sized berry of an evergreen tree native to Africa, West Indies, and Jamaica. It tastes like a combination of a number of aromatic spices.

Bouquet Garni: It is a small bundle of various fresh herbs. Traditionally it is composed of parsley, thyme, and bay leaf. This herb bundle gives stews, soups, or stocks an aromatic seasoning. The bouquet garni needs to be removed before serving the food.

Herbes de Provence: It is an assortment of dried herbs said to reflect those mostly commonly used in Southern France. The mixture commonly contains basil, fennel seed, lavender, marjoram, rosemary, sage, summer savory, thyme, and oregano.

Extracts: These are concentrated flavorings derived from various foods or plants usually through evaporation or distillation. They deliver a powerful flavor input to foods without adding excess volume or changing the consistency.

Chilies: (Capsicum annum) Red or green, are hot and add a spicy aromatic pungency to food. They are available fresh, dried, ground, pickled or in the form of paste or essence (extract). Chili peppers are of various kinds:

Jalapeño: Fairly hot green chilies, available bottled in brine or fresh from Specialty green-grocers

Small red Thai: Small, bright red and medium hot in flavor pepper.

Bird's eye Pepper: called Capsicum frutescens.

Habanero pepper: Red pepper

Serano: Red and long pepper

Espelette pepper: a variety of Capsicum annum (red chili). When using fresh peppers, it is advisable to remove the seeds which are the hottest part.

Seasoning cubes: They can be stock/bouillon cubes, meat, and chicken stock. The commonest of the cubes is the Maggi cube. It originated from Switzerland in 1886 by a Swiss German called Julius Maggi. This Maggi comes in sauce, granules, powder, paste, and cubes. The basic ingredients of maggi are salt, mono-sodium glutamate (MSG), spices, herbs, additives, and preservatives, hydrogenated vegetable fat. In Cameroon there is maggi in varied flavors of tomatoes, shrimps, beef, and chicken.

DIFFERENT DISHES AND BEST SPICES AND HERBS TO USE

BEEF	CHICKEN	FISH	PORK
Bay leaf	Basil	Bay leaf	Cayenne pepper
Basil	Bay leaf	Chives	Coriander
Cayenne pepper	Chives	Coriander	Curry powder
Cumin	Curry powder	Dill	Cumin
Curry powder	Coriander	Mustard	Dill
Garlic	Garlic	Sage	Garlic
Ginger	Ginger	Tarragon	Ginger
Marjoram	Marjoram	Thyme	Rosemary
Oregano	Oregano		Sage
Pepper	Thyme		Thyme
Thyme			
EGGS	**RICE**	**VEAL**	**LAMB**
Cayenne peppers	Chives	Bay leaf	Curry powder
Cumin	Cumin	Coriander	Dill
Curry powder	Curry powder	Dill	Garlic
Chives	Garlic	Garlic	Mint
Savory	Sage	Oregano	Oregano
Tarragon	Tarragon	Rosemary	Rosemary
		Sage	Thyme
		Thyme	
CARROTS	**SWEET PEPPER**	**AUBERGINES**	**MUSHROOMS**
Chives	Chives	Basil	Basil
Cumin	Coriander	Garlic	Chives
Ginger	Garlic	Marjoram	Dill
Marjoram	Marjoram	Oregano	Garlic
Mustard	Oregano	Pepper	Marjoram
Tarragon	Thyme	Sage	Oregano
		Thyme	Rosemary
			Tarragon
IRISH POTATOES	**DRY BEANS**	**TOMATOES**	**GREEN BEANS**

Bay leaf Chives Coriander Cumin Curry powder Dill Garlic	Cumin Cayenne pepper Coriander Garlic Marjoram Oregano Pepper	Chives Coriander Dill Garlic Marjoram Oregano Rosemary	Bay leaf Basil Dill Garlic Marjoram Mint
Mint Mustard Oregano Tarragon Thyme	Rosemary Sage Savory Tarragon Thyme	Sage Savory Tarragon Thyme	Rosemary Savory Tarragon
ZUCCHINI/SQUASH (COURGETTE)	**BEETROOT**	**PUMPKIN**	**BROCCOLI/ CABBAGE/ CAULIFLOWER/ BRUSSELS SPROUT**
Basil Dill Garlic Chives Mint Marjoram Tarragon	Caraway Chives Dill Ginger Horse radish	Bay leaf Cinnamon Cloves Curry powder Mace Mustard Rosemary Sage	Curry powder Cumin Basil Garlic Ginger Marjoram Oregano Tarragon Thyme
SEA FOOD	**SPINACH**	**PEAS**	**SWEET POTATOES**
Basil **Bay leaf** **Chervil** **Cloves** **Coriander** **Curry powder** **Dill** **Marjoram** **Oregano** **Tarragon** **Thyme**	**Basil** **Garlic** **Mustard** **Tarragon**	**Basil** **Chives** **Dill** **Marjoram** **Mint** **Oregano** **Savory** **Tarragon**	**Cinnamon** **Cloves** **Cayenne pepper** **Muscat**

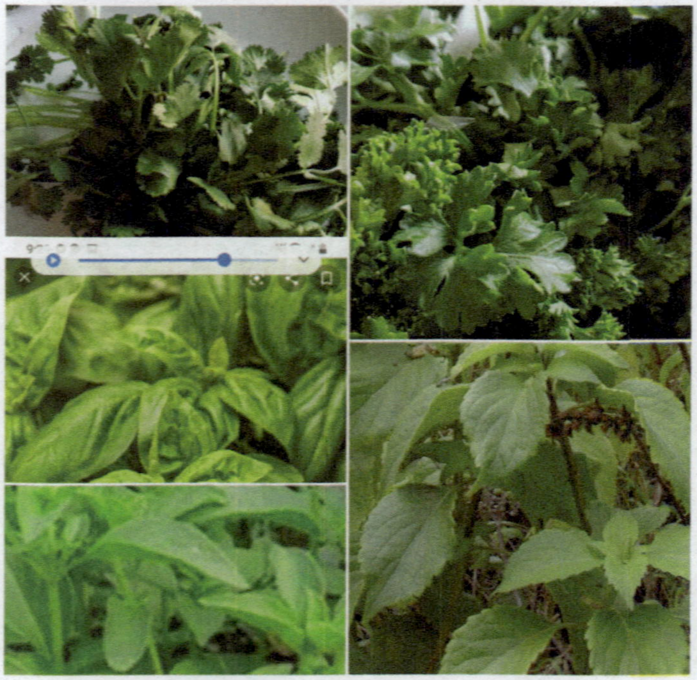

Coriander, parsley, basil, wild basil (kotmanji), African basil (masepu, massep)

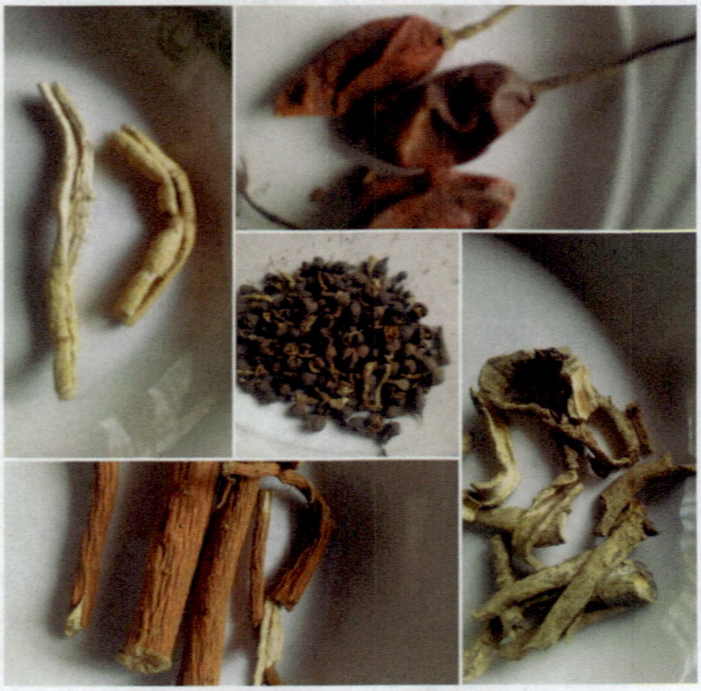

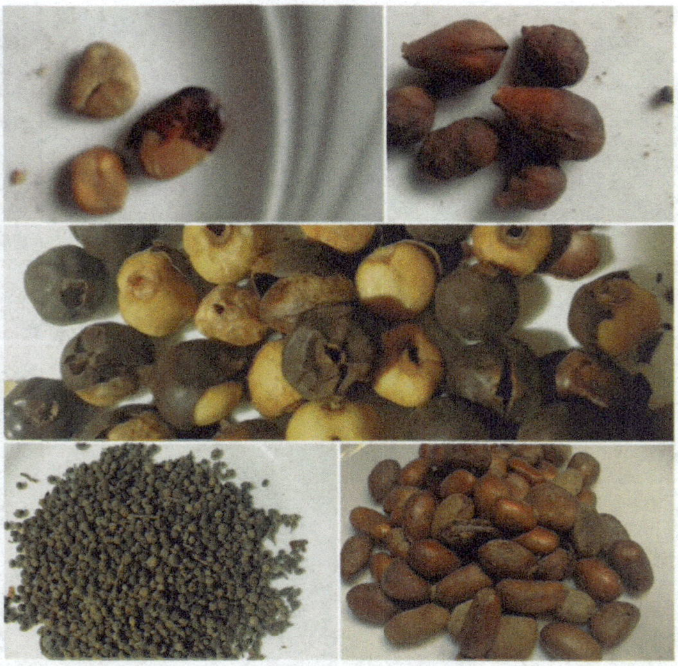

Nkwi spices

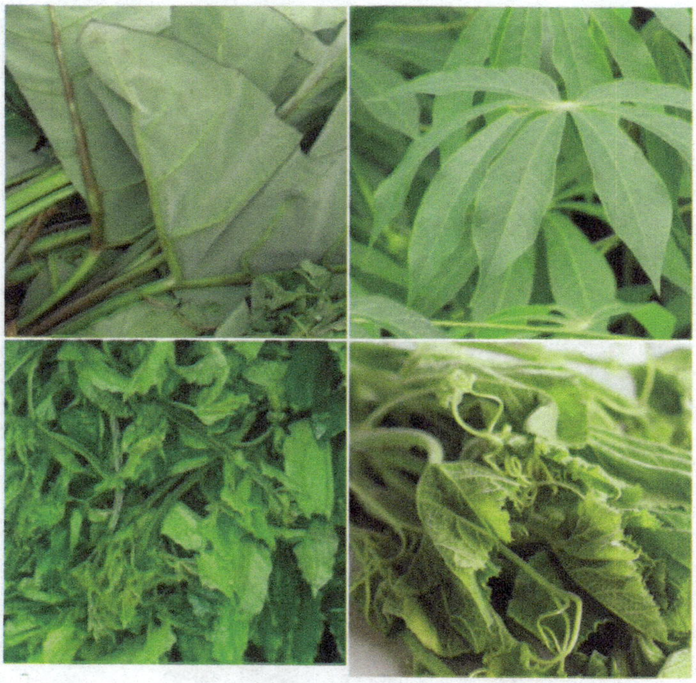

Cocoyam (taro) leaves, cassava leaves, fluted pumpkin leaves (okongobong), pumpkin leaves.

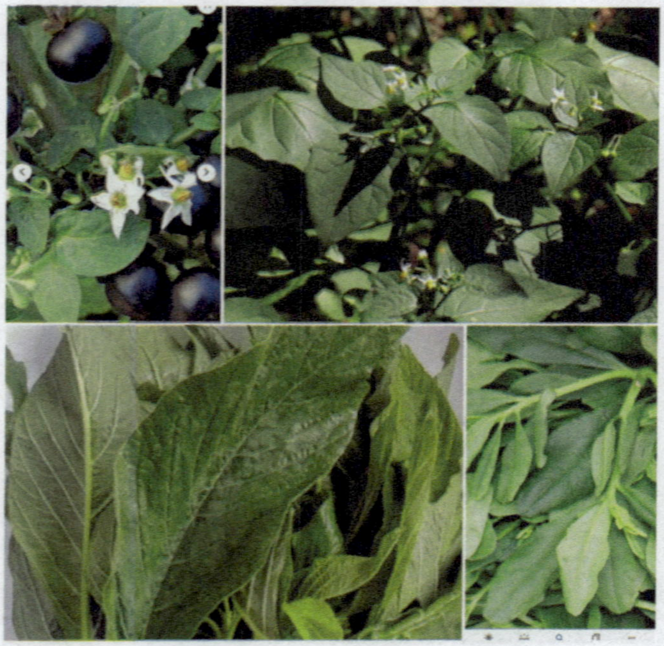

Night shade leaves (huckleberry leaves, njama-njama), amaranth (green), water leaves.

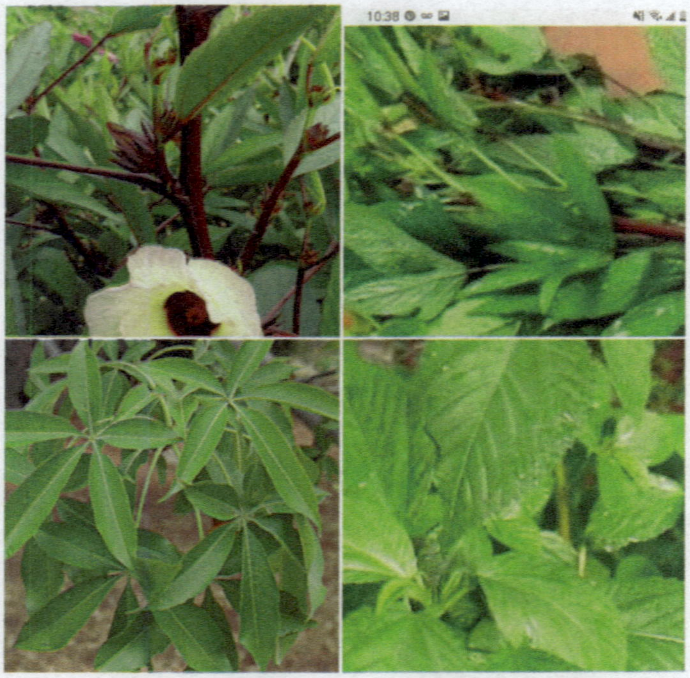

Sour leaves (roselle), baobab leaves, jute mallow leaves

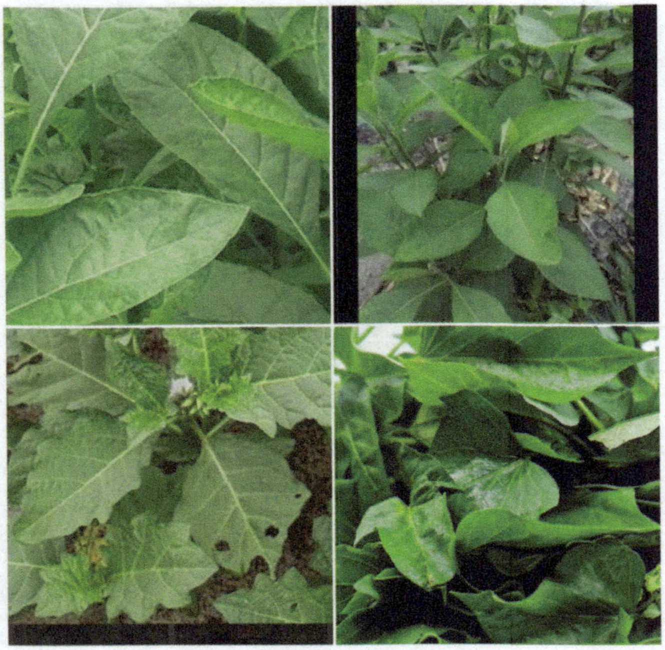

Bitterleaves, garden egg leaves (anchia), sweet potato leaves.

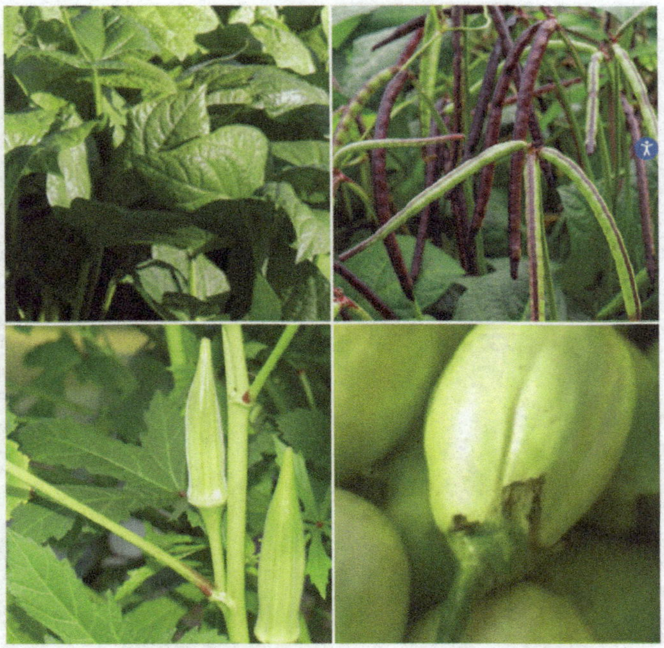

Cow pea leaves (waah), cow fresh cow peas, okro leaves and fruit, African garden eggs (njagatu)

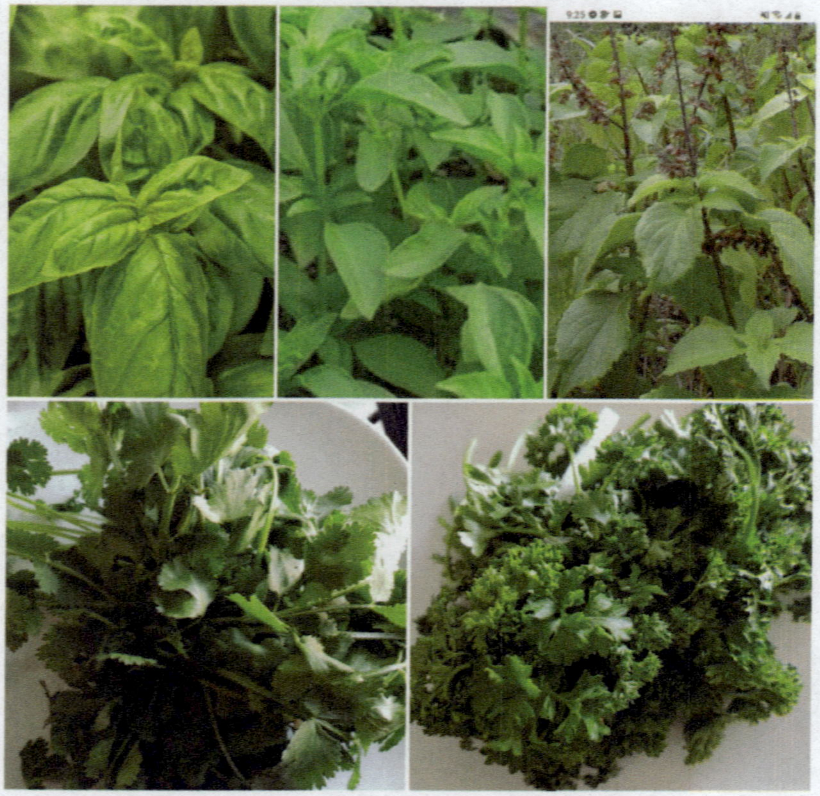

Basil, African basil (cutmargin), wild basil (masepo/masep), coriander, parsley.

THE FOOFOO DISH

The foofoo is a specialty dish from Cameroon and other West African countries. This dish is prepared from the staple foods of cassava, cocoyams, colocasia, yams, maize, rice, millet, plantains, and sorghum. The dish is eaten with all types of soups, thin and thick soups, vegetables, stews, and sauces. The foofoo can be called fufu, fufuo, foufou, or couscous. Foofoo is prepared in two ways such as:

The starchy tubers such as cassava, yams, cocoyams, etc. are boiled in water and pounded briskly using a mortar and pestle into a white pliable and sticky dough-like consistency.

The flour of some of the starchy foods such as maize, cassava, yams etc. are poured into boiling water and stirred vigorously to avoid lumps forming. It is then cooked into a soft paste. It is eaten best when still hot. A bit of the fufu is formed into eatable balls, dipped in the soup, and swallowed.

FOO FOO DISHES: Corn foo foo, cooked water foofoo, garri foofoo, kwangkalang, akwa a, kwa' a, Couscous de maïs, Foufou de riz, Couscous de manioc, Foo foo d'igname, Boules d'igname, Foo foo de garri.

COLOCACIA DISHES

ACHU FOOFOO

The achu foofoo is food of the Ngemba people, and some people of Tikari descend of the North West Region of Cameroon, and some Bamileke people of the West Region of Cameroon. Apart from the Bali Chambas of Mezam Division, all inhabitants of this Division have this prestigious dish as their traditional meal which is eaten at every important occasion.

An achu dish is a whitish paste made from a combination of three varieties of cocoyams; colocasia esculenta known locally as taro or Ibo, Colocasia Xanthosoma sagittifolium known locally as macabo, whose mains are called "mamie cocoyam," and a variety of bananas called the dwarf banana is sometimes added at will.

The dwarf banana is used in achu because of many reasons. First it is softer than any other banana and thus easier to pound. Secondly the banana adds bulk to the cocoyams, reduces its carbohydrate content, reduces the elasticity of some cocoyams, and hardens soft cocoyams. In addition, its nutritious values are not to be under-estimated.

The cocoyam for achu is a rich source of energy, calcium, and iron. The ingredients are usually cooked in the jacket and then peeled while they are still hot to make pounding easier. It takes two or more people to prepare this dish. Some people peel while others pound, but with modern technology an individual can do it with a heavy fruit juicer to grind the cocoyams and bananas. The finished product is an elastic, whitish and sticky paste.

The achu fufu by itself is not delicious and has a bland taste. The soup with which it is eaten is what makes this dish the "caviar" of the Bamenda people in particular, and the country in general. The yellow soup is the typical soup that traditionally goes with achu. The yellow soup is made from palm oil, emulsified with potash, or limestone, a salt-like rock or powder base called kanwa or sel gemme. Traditionally unripen green plantain peelings are dried, burnt and processed in a manner to have a residual ash which, when dissolved in water acts as the kanwa. This ash residue is called "nikie" in the Ngemba dialect.

There is also the black soup whose main ingredient is the cocoyam leaves of the colocasia esculenta. The young leaves are harvested, cooked, and dried to be used for the soup. The leaves, which are best used, are those from the green or pink stems of Ibo cocoyams and the leaves from the red Xanthosoma sagittifolium which is the red cocoyam leaves. Other leaves not in this category have calcium oxalate which irritates the throat, commonly known as the throat scratching when eaten. This black soup is called "ndza ati-tii" in Ngemba. The fresh or dried cocoyam leaves are called "abangee," "ambaa," or "ateeb" all in the Ngemba dialect. In addition to the leaves, sometimes the blossoms of the cocoyams are used in place of the cocoyam leaves. The blossom has a very delicious aroma. It is called "ataree" or "antweree' in the Bafut and Mankon dialects. If the blossom is used the soup will not be as black as the soup from the leaves. The cocoyam leaves are rich in vitamin A, B1, B2, and C

No matter which kind of soup is used to eat achu, the soup will be cooked with a variety of meats such as beef skin, usually called kanda or Katanga, beef tripe called towel, entrails, fresh or smoked beef, smoked or fresh game, smoked fish especially, and catfish called mud fish. Oxtail, trotters of beef called foot cow are also other varieties of meat used. Many spices are used in preparing the achu soup, but the original traditional spices are just three: the African or Ethiopian pepper called "kiengi," West African called "sopp", and birds eye peppers called "tita sing."

There is something that makes this dish special and that is its accompaniments which include boiled or roast Africsn garden eggs, sautéed huckleberry leaves called "njama-njama," boiled mushrooms called "nboh" or "kokobiako," crushed boiled young elephant shoot called "asisong" or "funisongnuï", and egusi pudding. Sometimes fresh or dried cooked garden eggs are used to thicken the soup.

This special dish is eaten with one finger, the forefinger of the righthand. The paste has a trough in the middle where the soup is put. Eating is from the outside inward avoiding the breaking of the trough thus preventing soup from flowing out. Traditionally, it is eaten from the banana leaf in which achu is normally wrapped although plates are used nowadays. In the days gone-by it was a family meal whereby the family gathered to eat from a big bundle of achu.

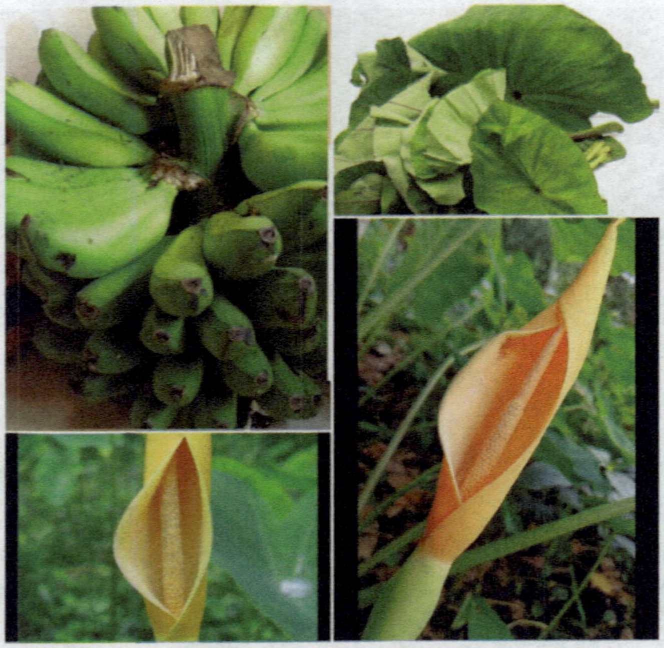

Achu bananas, taro leaves, taro blossom or flowers.

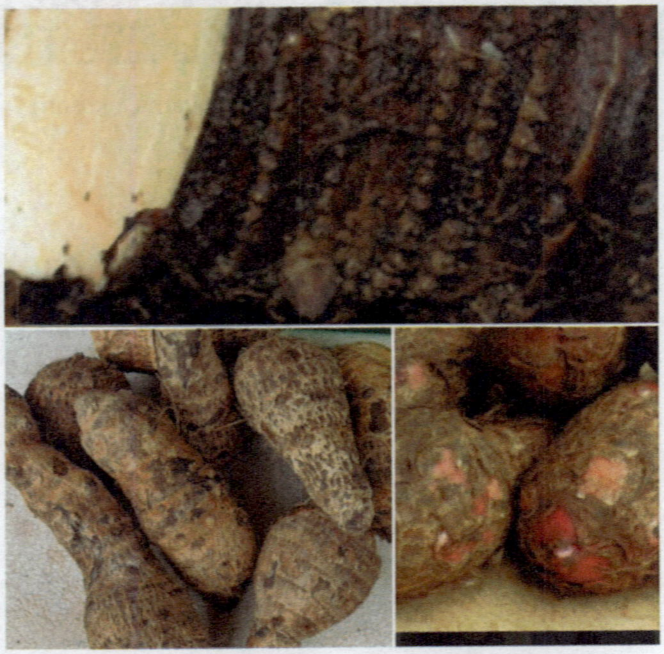

Xanthosoma sagittifolium. (macabo, malanga)

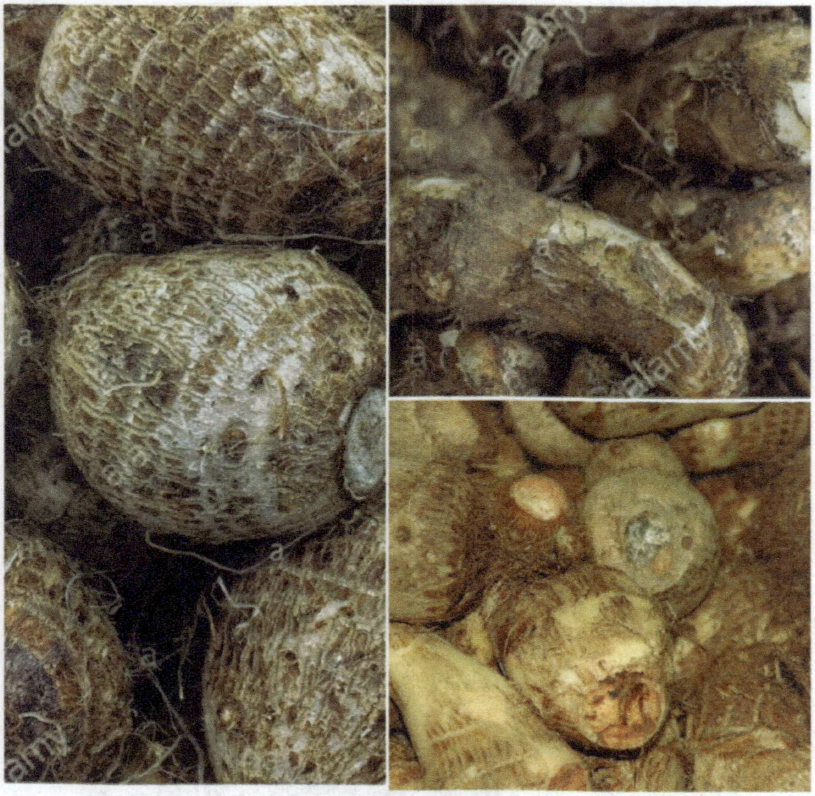

Colocasia antiquorium (country cocoyams, nku-uh)

YELLOW ACHU SOUP

- Ndzaa Nikie is the Ngemba version of Achu Soup
- Ndzaa funüsongnü is elephant grass shoots soup Ngemba style.
- Yellow soup with African eggplant is Bamileke style of yellow soup using fresh African
- eggplant. The use of dry African eggplant is special to Bafut of Mezam, Division version.
- Chi na'a yellow soup with okro is a Bamileke version of yellow soup.

YELLOW ACHU SOUP SPICES

1.	Tetrapleura tetraptera:	Fruit of aridan tree, Eseke-seke
2.	Monodora myristica:	Calabash nutmeg, Pébè, nding
3.	Echinops giganteus:	Globe thistle, soapte, kahgoh, tchamngne, tsegum, kessa
4.	Afrostyrax lepidophyllus:	Fruit of garlic tree, country onion, foulom, bush onion.
5.	Capsicum frutescens:	Bird's eye pepper, jalapeno pepper, chili pepper
*6.	Piper guineese:	Bush pepper, West African pepper, sopp, jowe, uziza pepper, Thai pepper
7.	Fogara leprierii:	Odoriferous grapes, prickly ash
8.	Fagara xanthoxyloides:	Open mouth, Sichuan pepper, ngachu'u, Chinese coriander, natchou
9.	Pentadeplanda brazzeana:	White liang
*10.	Xylopia aethiopica:	Ethiopian pepper, kiengi, bikwi, kili pepper

NB: * Are the most important spices for the yellow Achu Soup.

COCOYAM TUBER DISHES

Nku-uh pottage: It is a colocasia antiquorium pottage of the Ngemba ethnic group of Mezam Division in the North West Region of Cameroon.

Macabo ma sese: It is a Douala style pottage cocoyams.

Mpélé macab: is Bamileke style pottage cocoyams.

Cocoyam pottage: cooked in meat and smoked fish North West and South West style.

Bende Na Erembi: It is an Iroko (Ndian, South West Region) dish consisting of boiled cocoyams (Bende) with cocoyam leaves (Erembi)

GRATED COCOYAM DISHES

The cocoyam tuber of the baby Xanthosoma sagittifolium called macabo, is one of the main staple food stuffs of Cameroon. It is cooked in varied ways throughout the Republic. One of the cherished methods is by grating and mixing it with spices and steamed or boiled as delicious dishes.

Equacoco à vekoo: (Endeley bread) is a dish of the Bakweri ethnic group of Buea, Fako Division of South West Region. The traditional name is Kwacoco Bible.

Equacoco: (Equan) ya mosaka is also a Bakweri dish of grated cocoyams (equacoco or equan) eaten with mbanga soup or palm nut soup called mosaka (ngonya mosaka) or any other preferred soup.

Ekwang: It is grated cocoyam pottage of the Oroko ethnic group of Ndian Division of the South West Region of Cameroon.

Kouakoukou: It is grated cocoyam, Bamileke style

Bekwong: It is a Bassa and Beti dish, ethnic groups of Centre and South Regions, similar to the equacoco à vekoo.

Bekwong au feuilles de macabo: It is a koki, the same as simple bekwong except with the addition of cocoyam leaves and more palm oil.

Bekwan: It is a Douala dish same as Bekwong.

Macabo rape: It is a grated cocoyam dish with the addition of roast groundnuts.

Timba na busa: It is equacoco tossed in palm nut soup (sese equan ya mosaka).

COCOYAM LEAF SOUPS

Ndzaa atii-tii: It is commonly called black soup used for eating the achu fufu.

Macabo cocoyam leaf soup: It is cooked with egusi, smoked fish, beef, crayfish, and other ingredients.

Ebeb Lombo: 1 &2 is a Beti name for soup cooked with young cocoyam leaves

Baombe soup: It is cooked with cocoyam leaves

Soupe achu noire: Black soup.

Ragout: de feuilles de macabo rouge.

Esuba soup: A saltless soup of cocoyam leaves, dish of the Bakossi ethnic group of Kupe Manenguba division, South West Region.

Erembi: is cocoyam leaf soup of the Iroko people of Ndian Division of South West Region of Cameroon.

CASSAVA TUBER DISHES

Cassava batons or chikwangues: (miondo & bobolo)

Miondo (Baton de manioc-fins grains) is a 25cm long, 2cm wide cassava paste of the Douala people. Bobolo (Bebebolo) – batons de manioc gros grains is a baguette shape of about 30cm long, 5cm wide of cassava paste of the people of the Centre and South Regions of Cameroon.

Antégue-kouma: It is a cassava purée of the people of the East Region of Cameroon.

Mbōn–lep: It is cooked cassava, steeped in water and washed. A useful way to serve left-over cooked cassava as an aperitif. A dish of the villages of the South Region of Cameroon.

Gateau de manioc: is cassava koki.

Masoma: It is a cassava snack of the North West and South West Regions of Cameroon, and the Republic of Nigeria. Cassava is cooked, steeped in water, and washed and eaten with coconut as a snack. It is the same as Mbon-lep.

Mintumba: It is a cassava koki made of fermented cassava. A dish of the inhabitants of Bafia and Bassa of the Central Region of Cameroon.

Soya bean mintumba: Mintumba is enriched with soya bean

Ekok'a Makwamba: It is a cassava koki of the Douala people of the Littoral Region of Cameroon.

Cassava koki: It is mixture of grated cassava, and other ingredients tied in plantain leaves and steamed.

Manioc à l'huile: (koki de manioc): Same as cassava koki.

Mkonda: It is a dish of cassava paste and roast groundnuts. (Cassava koki)

IRISH POTATO DISHES

Pounded Irish potatoes Mix: with red or black beans

Green pepper/Irish potato pottage

Curry Irish potatoes: Are parboiled Irish potatoes, coated with curry powder, and fried.

Irish potatoes galettes: is grated Irish potatoes mixed with flour, eggs and other ingredients and fried.

Fried Irish Potatoes: Are potatoes peeled and sliced into batonnets, not washed but wiped and fried in oil three times.

Irish potato pottage: It is pottage in which coconut milk is added. It is sometimes called "poto poto" Irish which means "mud-mud" because it is cooked until soft and blended with all the other ingredients.

Plain Boiled Irish potatoes: Are peeled potatoes boiled in water, bay leaf and onions.

MAIZE DISHES

Corn chaff: It is a typical dish of the North West Region of Cameroon. It is beans and corn pottage in palm oil be it fresh beans and fresh corn or dried beans and dried corn with the addition of spices.

Corn koki: It is milled fresh corn mixed with ingredients and palm oil, tied in plantain leaves, and steamed.

Fresh corn purée: It is fresh corn, spinach and garden eggs cooked in oil until soft.

Corn koki: is the South Region of Cameroon version of the North West corn koki. Fresh ground corn mixed in oil, tied.

Maize galette: It is fresh corn grains mixed with maizena, eggs, and other ingredients and fried.

Fresh corn and fresh groundnut koki: are when these two ingredients, are mixed with shrimps, oil, and other ingredients, wrapped in plantain leaves, and steamed.

Ekomba: is fresh or dried corn mixed with dried groundnuts ground into a paste, tied in bundles, and steamed.

Corn pudding (Abolo): is cooked foofoo mixed with corn meal and wheat flour, or grated sweet potatoes let it rise, and then steamed in plantain leaves.

Le Sanga: is fresh corn grains and zom leaves cooked in palmnut jus. It is a pottage of South Region.

Le Sanga'a met à Mboa: is fresh corn spiced with hiomi, sésang leaves or ba'am cooked in palm oil.

Corn tchap: is Bamileke version of corn chaff.

THE PAP MEAL

Pap is a gruel made from either fresh or dried corn, rice, millet, or sorghum. Corn pap is made by soaking the corn grains for some days, depending on the state of the corn and the climate. The grains are strained off of water and ground to a wet paste. This paste is soaked in water, washed, and sieved. The chaff is removed, and the liquid is allowed to settle. This liquid is decanted and cooked to a paste called pap. The name pap depends on the starting material e.g., corn pap from corn, millet pap from millet, and fresh corn pap from fresh corn.

The pap can be fortified with many ingredients such as milk, eggs, crayfish, groundnut paste, fruit juice, fish powder, bean powder and sugar or honey to sweeten it.

Pap is the first weaning dish for Cameroonian children, a favorable dish for patients and invalids, lactating mothers and for Moslems who break their fast after a day's fasting.

PAP DISHES

Rice water, corn pap, corn flour pap, fresh corn pap, hausa foofoo pap, groundnut/corn pap, Bouillie de mil, Bouillie de maïs Camerounaise, Bouillie de mil au soja, Bouillie de petite mil for infants of 4-6 months, Eau de riz, Semoule de maïs, Bouillie fine, Bouillie de maïs et arachide, Koukoulou, and bouille de mais.

RICE DISHES

Coconut rice: is rice cooked with chicken, smoked fish or pork cooked in coconut milk.

Fried rice: is long grain rice cooked with beef, liver gizzard or kidneys, **Jollof rice pottage, Fried rice pottage, Buea style jollof rice is a type of coconut rice, Riz sauté are other rice.**

PLANTAIN DISHES

Onganven: It is a mixture of uncooked ripe and raw plantains pounded with raw ground groundnuts into a paste and tied in plantain leaves and steamed by the Bulu and Ewondo people of the Centre Region of Cameroon. It is known as ripe plantain koki

Pounded ripe plantain and beans mix: is a favorite of the Western Region.

Ripe plantain koki is pounded ripe plantain: mixed with fish and palm oil and tied in plantain leaves and steamed.

Plantain and pork are a pottage: of the Ngemba style of Mezam Division of the North West Region of Cameroon.

Ntouba Ekon: is pounded green plantains or partially ripe plantains and eaten with egusi soup by the Bulus, the Betis of the South, Centre Regions, and the Doulas of the Littoral Region.

Ndengué: is a thick purée of cooked mix ripe and unripe plantains pounded and cooked into a purée. It is eaten with a soup by the people of the East Region.

Sese plantains: is a pottage of the North West and South West people cooked with beef and palm oil.

Kondré: is a plantain pottage, a Bamileke specialty.

Banane malaxée: is banana pottage cooked with raw groundnut paste.

Mekere Na erembi: is a dish of boiled plantains and cocoyam leaf soup of the Oroko ethnic group of Ndian Division of the South West Region.

Mekere Na ndondi: is boiled plantains eaten with fish.

Mekere Na Ndonga: is boiled plantains eaten with pepper paste.

Mekere Na ndoh: is boiled plantains eaten with bitter leaves.

Mekere Na ndondi Na ebonge: is boiled plantains eaten with boiled fresh fish and broad leaf vegetables, a traditional leaf.

VEGETABLES

The Northwest and West Regions of Cameroon are the bread baskets of vegetables and green herbs in the Republic of Cameroon. Other regions produce some vegetables, mostly for local consumption within the regions. The root vegetables are frequently eaten because they can be prepared into foofoo and eaten with the leafy vegetables. Some vegetables such as broccoli, asparagus, cauliflower, courgette, aubergines, and beet roots are still not well present in the Cameroon cuisine.

Carrots, green beans, bitterleaves, okro fruit and leaves, cassava leaves, pumpkin leaves, cabbages, tomatoes, and onions are the predominant vegetables found in diets of most homes. Some of the vegetables are cooked during special occasions and most often they are used as garnishes. Njama-njama is the simplest vegetable in the country. It is the main vegetable soup used for people who eat corn foofoo. It has many varieties such as green stems, purple stems, small leaves, and broad leaves. It is known by varied names throughout the country such as huckleberry leaves, country njama-njama, ndhza-nkang, njapsheun, mbas and zom, etc.

SN	English name	French name	Scientific name	Common name
1	Asparagus	Asperge	Asparagus officinalis	
2.	Aubergine	Aubergine	Solanum spp	Garden eggs Eggplant
3.	African eggplant	Aubergine Africaine	Solanum aethiopicum L.	African eggplant Garden eggs Scarlet eggplant Djagaturu (Bakossi) Nyoh (Banganté) Cheuche (Dschang) Zong (Eton, Bulu, Ewondo) Nga (Bamoun) Hisingui (Bassa) Gaouta (Hausa) Anyére (Ngemba) Gijo Njakatu

4.	African eggplant leaves	Feuilles d'aubergine d'Africiane	Solanum macracarpon L.	African eggplant leaves Big nightshades Gboma eggplant Ornamental eggplant leaves Ndjapkieh (Bangangté) Nyen baa bitodo (Bassa) Etoé (Bulu) Nkéa (Douala) Ntondo (Eton) Anguko (Fufuldé) Ngago (Hausa) Anchia (North West)
5.	Baobab leaves	Feuilles de baobab Pain de singe (fruit) Arbre aux calebasses Arbre de mille ans Calebassier du Senegal	Adansonia digitata	Monkey breadtree Ethiopian sourgourd Cream of tartar tree Senegal calabash fruit Upside-down tree
6.	Beetroot	Betteraves	Beta vulgaris	
7.	Bitterleaf	Feuille amère	Vernonia amygdalina	Ndole Ndola Douala N'dole Nying (Ngemba) Nyii (Bafut)
8.	Black-eye pea leaves	Feuille de pois	Vigna unguiculata	Cow pea leaves Wagu (Ngemba) Waah (Bali)
9.	Broccoli	Chou-fleur	Brassica oleracea	-
10.	Cabbage	Chou	Brassica oleracea	-
11.	Cassava leaf	Feuille de manioc	Manihot utilissima	-
12.	Cocoyam leaf	Feuille de macabo rouge (Redcocoyan leaves) Ibo cocoyam leaves Country cocoyam leaves (Nkwuh)	Xanthosoma sagittifolium Colocasia esculenta Colocasiaantiqcorium	Ateb Abanga Ngemba Ambaa (Bafut) Mbongéré (Bakweri) Balumdji (Fufuldé Baombe
13.	Cocoyam blossom (flower)	Fleur de taro	Colocasia esculenta	Atare (Bafut) Antere (Ngemba)
14.	Carrot	Carotte	Daucus carota	
15.	cauliflower	Chou-fleur	Brassica oleracea	-
16.	Chinese cabbage	Chou-Chinios	Brassica spp	-
17.	Cucumber	Concombre	Cucumis sativus	-

18.	Courgette	Courgette	Cicurbita pepo	Zucchini Squash Marrow (UK, Ireland) Baby marrows (S.A.)
19.	Cow pea leaf	Feuille de haricot	Palmate doux	Wagu (Ngemba) Waah (Bali)
20.	Elephant grass shoots	Herbe à l'éléphant	Pennisetum Purpureaum	Funüsongnu (Ngemba) Assissong Minsong Vekoko Fureusongni (Bafut)
21.	Fluted pumpkin leaf	Feuille de courge	Telfairia occidentalis	Ekongobong Gourd
22.	Green beans	Haricot vert	Phaseolus vulgaris	String beans Snap beans French beans French green beans
23.	Nightshades	Feuille d'airelle	Evo yora cocohorus Solanum scabrum S. villorsum	Ndhza nkang (Ngemba) Njama-njama (N.W. R) Njap lah (Bamileke) Wosangu (Bakweri) Ba'am (Bassa) Zom (Bulu, Ewondo) Bitosso (Bafia) Koumbi/Hakondjam (Fufulde) Kolinski (Hausa) Huckleberry leaves
			Dwarf tamarillo Cyphomandra abutiloide seeds	Tree tomatoes
24.	Jute mallow	Feuille gluante	Corchorus olitorius L. C Tridens L C Trilocularis L	Keleng-keleng (Douala) Lalo (Fufulde) Tegue (Bulu, Ewondo) Gbarak (Bafia) Teuere messi (Bamoun Django (Bassa) Nkeleng (Bamileke) Cren-crean (NWR)
25.	Lettuce	Laitue	Latuca sativa	-
26.	Mushroom	Champignon	Agarius sp	Nboh Njojo Kokobiako

27.	Okro leaf	Feuille de gombo	Hibiscus esculentus	Nzeng Akagang (Ngemba)
28.	Okro fruit	Gombo	Abelmoschus esculentus	Pés (Eton) Bitetam (Bulu, Ewondo) Akro (Bamileke) Gbarack à budum (Bafia) Ha (Bamoun) Bascode (Fufuldé) Koye (Bassa) Kigang (Douala) Koubeowa (Hausa) Lady's fingers Gumbo
29.	Pumpkin leaf	Feuille de potiron	Cucurbita pepo	Nzeng Nibo (Ngemba)
30.	Pumpkin	Courge	Cucurbita pepo	Potiron Liwove Niboh (Ngemba)
31.	Sour leaf	Feuille amère	Solanum negro	-
32.	Spinach	Epinard	Spinacia oleracea	Bush green
33.	Sweet pepper	Poivron	Capsicum annum	Bell pepper Capsicum Jon's head A pepper (UK, Canada)
34.	Sweet potato leaf	Feuille de patate	Ipomoea batatas	Dankari (Fulfudé) Andonge (Bafut)
35.	Tomato	Tomate	Lycopersicum esculentum	Plante de tomate
36.	Water leaf	Feuille d'eau	Tatinum triangulare	Bush spinach Wild spinach
37	Chayotte	Chayotte	Sechiumrdule	Miritton, Vegetable peas Chocho Christophims Sayote Chayote Squash

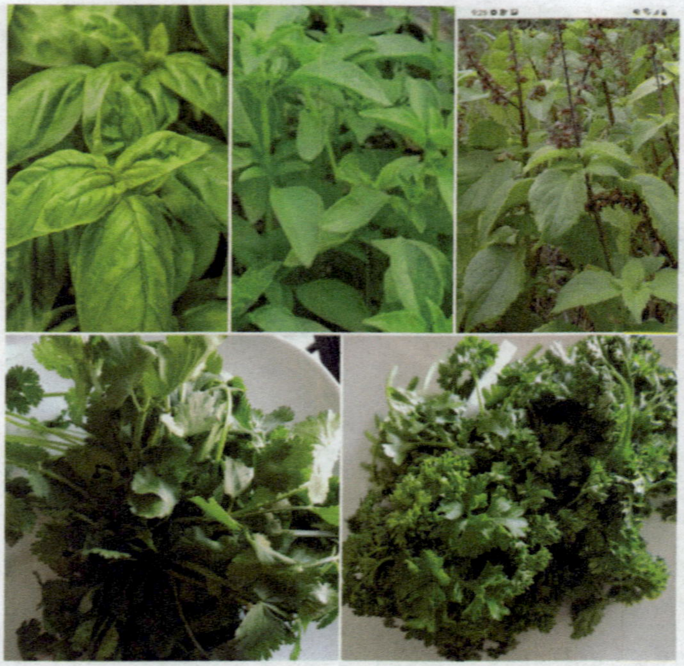

Basil, African basil (cutmargin), wild basil (masepo/masep), coriander, parsley.

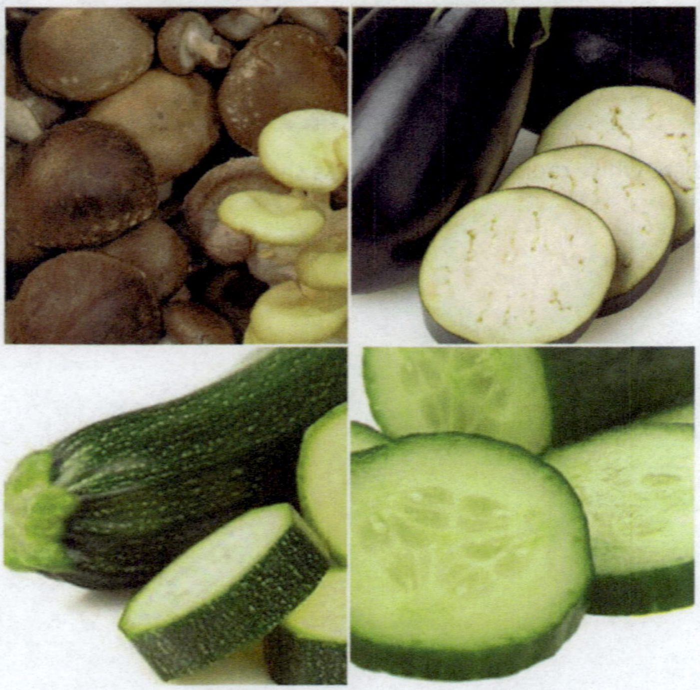

Mushrooms (kokobiako, iboh), aubergine, courgette, cucumber

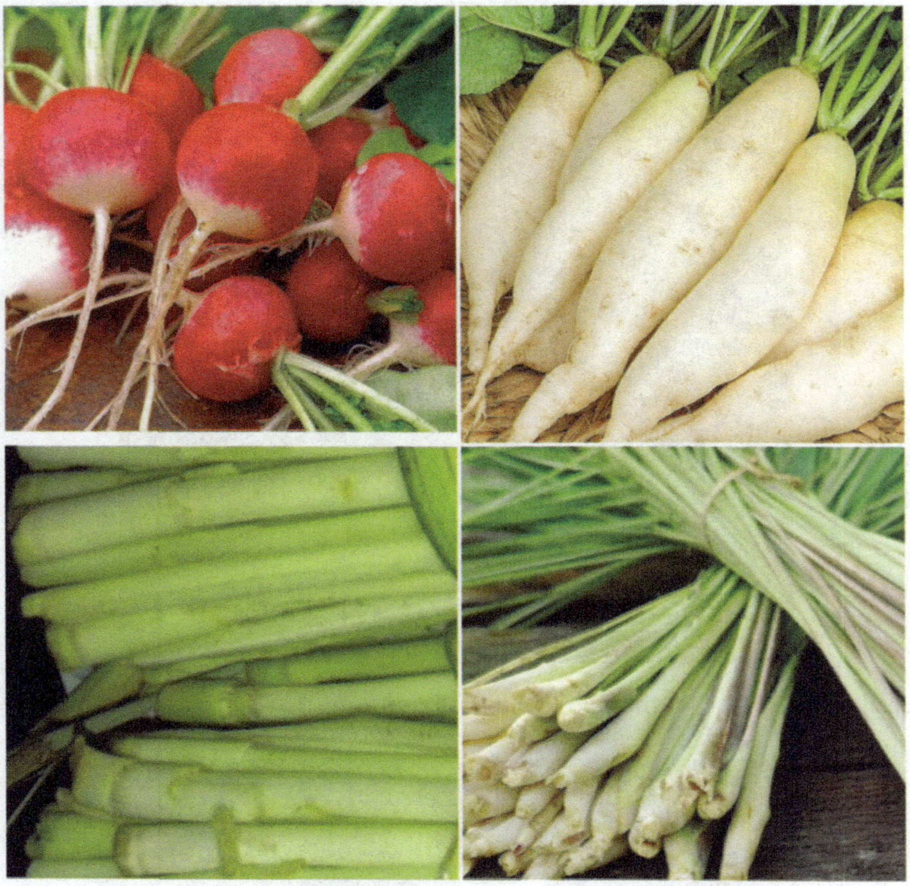

Red radish, white radish, elephant grass shoots, lemon grass (fever grass)

VEGETABLE DISHES

Vegetable pottage, sautéed cucumber, Irish potato curry, carrots glazed in five spices, spiced cauliflower, red cabbage curry, sautéed sweet peppers, vegetable curry, Provence pottage, braised beetroot in vinegar, grated courgette paste, Bordelaise mushroom, good woman pottage, courgettes sauté à vinaigre, sauté carrots an Irish potatoes, Ratatouille, glazed carrots and orange.

"AMARANTUS" LEAVES

SCIENTIFIC NAMES: Amarantus cruentus, A. Lividsu, A. dubius

COMMON NAMES: Amaranth, pigweed, green

LOCAL NAMES:

Kumkum (Bafia), Biwolé (Bewolé) (Douala), Ndjap mekat (Banganté), Agnaka/Hakondjam (Fulfudé), Feufe (Dschang), Gagnorwa (Hausa), Teue (Bamoun), Kumkuma (Eton), Po'oga (Bassa), Green (North West and South West Regions), Folong (Bulu, Ewondo), Fii (Ngemba, Mezam Division)

BITTERLEAF DISHES

Bitterleaf is a vegetable whose botanical name is **Vernonia amydalina**. It is a bitter herb related to chicory, sometimes used as a quinine substitute for malaria and other illnesses with high fever. Bitterleaf is mentioned in the Book of Exodus 12:8. Dandelion is one of the bitter herbs eaten at the Passover. The twigs of bitterleaf shrubs are a favorite chewing stick for dental and oral hygiene.

Bitterleaves are known by different names in different countries. In Cameroon it is called ndolé, ndoh or just bitterleaf. Grawa in Amharic (Ethiopia), Eworu in Yoruba (Nigeria), etidot in Ibibio (Nigeria) Onugu in Ibo (Nigeria), ityuna in Tiv (Nigeria), chusa-doki in Hausa, mululuza (Lugarda), cabwori in Acholi, olusia in Luo, Nying in Ngemba. It is cooked using different methods and ingredients throughout the country and can also be used as vegetables in pottages.

BITTERLEAF SOUPS

Ndolé soup: It is bitterleaf cooked in groundnut paste, tomato and meat or smoked fish. It is a specialty of the Douala people of Cameroon

Bitterleaf soup: It is a soup cooked with bitter leaves and egusi with fish such as stock fish and / or smoked kuta or shine nose fish.

Soya bean vernonia soup: Bitterleaves cooked and enriched with soya bean paste and beef.

Shrimp / meat ndole soup: Ndole cooked with fresh beef and fresh shrimps.

Shrimp ndole soup: Bitterleaves cooked with beef and dried shrimps (crayfish).

Le ndolé aux crevettes 1 as number 5 above.

Ndolé à la viande aux crevettes 2 as number 4 above.

Sauce de vernonia au soja: Bitterleaves soup enriched in soya bean paste.

CASSAVA LEAF DISHES

Saltless kpwem (kpwem sans sel): A saltless cassava leaf soup of the Beti people of the Centre and South Regions of Cameroon. Cooked in palm nut jus, ripe bananas and aubergines.

Beef in cassava leaves: Cassava leaf cooked with beef and roast groundnut paste.

Mbom kpwen: a Beti dish of cassava leaves pounded, mixed with soya bean and other ingredients, tied in plantain leaves, and steamed.

Cassava leaf soup: Cassava leaf cooked in palm oil, onions, and salt. A Democratic Republic of Congo dish.

Cassava leaf soup: Beef, groundnuts, smoked fish, and other ingredients are used to cook this soup.

Boeuf aux feuilles de manioc: A soup cooked with cassava leaves, beef, roast groundnuts, and palm oil.

NIGHT SHADE LEAVES

SCIENTIFIC NAMES: Solanum scabrum, S. villorsum, Night shades

COMMON NAMES: Garden huckleberry, huckleberry leaves, njama-njama

LOCAL NAMES: Zom: (Bulu, Ewondo), Njaplah (Bamileke), Ba'am (Bassa), Bitosso (Bafia), Djaptcheun (Bamoun), Koumbi/ Hakondjam (Fufuldé), Kolinski (Hausa), Njama-njama (North West Region), Wosangu (Bakweri – South West Region), Ndzha-nkang, ambore, nyuyseji, mbas (North West names) Huckleberry leaves are leaves from a shrub almost similar to the spinach. This shrub produces blue to violet seeds which are not consumed as food. Some nightshade fruits, the dwarf tamarillo is consumed and known in Cameroon as Tree tomato. There are many varieties of the nightshade leaves in Cameroon - big leaves called Foumbot or Bamoun njama-njama, small leaves called Banso njama-njama, medium leaves, purple stems, green steams, bitter and bitterless types coming from various villages of the North West Region of Cameroon especially Babanki or Kejem Ketingoh. At first taste it is bitter, but as any guest gets used to it, it becomes a favorite vegetable. When you hear of country njama-njama it is the nightshade.

The nightshade vegetables in Yaounde is the big leaves. It is called zom by the Ewondo and Bulu people. The bitter and bitterless varieties are available.

NIGHT SHADE LEAF DISHES

Njama-njama leaf soup It is a soup of huckleberry leaves known in the North West Region of Cameroon as njama-njama or plain njama-njama or country njama-njama. It is sometimes cooked saltless by the Kom and Nso people of the North West Region.

Wosangu soup is the Bakweri style of cooking huckleberry leaves with egusi and smoked fish.

Ossang is soup of zom leaves and egusi of the kaka and mbaya people of the East Region of Cameroon.

Meukeleu is zom leaves and groundnut paste of the Kaka and Mbaya people of the East Region of Cameroon tied in plantain leaves and steamed.

Zom non amèr au soja is soup cooked with feuilles de zom non amèr in soya beans powder by the Ewondo people of the Centre Region of Cameroon

Nightshade leaves with African Eggplant is a traditional dish of the Beti people of the Centre and South Regions of Cameroon cooked with palm nut jus. It is greatly appreciated by the elderly.

N'dzap is a typical dish of the Dschang people of Menoua division of Bamileke ethnic group of West Region of Cameroon involving sautéed nightshade.

THE AFRICAN EGGPLANT AND LEAVES

EGGPLANT (FRUIT)

SCIENTIFIC NAME: Solanum aethiopicum L

COMMON NAMES: African eggplant, garden eggs, scarlet eggplant.

LOCAL NAMES: Djagaturu (Bakossi), Nyoh (Bangangte, Zong (Eton, Ewondo, Bulu), Nga (Bamoun), Hisingui (Bassa), Gaouta (Hausa), Njakatu (Pidgin English)

Anyere (Ngemba), Aubergine (French)

AFRICAN EGGPLANT LEAVES

SCIENTIFIC NAME: Solanum macrocarpan L

COMMON NAMES: African eggplant, big nightshades, gboma eggplant, ornamental Eggplant.

LOCAL NAMES: Ndzap kieh (Bangante), Nyen baa bitodo (Bassa), Etoe (Bulu)

Nkea (Douala), Ntonda (Eton), Anguko (fulfulde), Ngago (Hausa),

Anchia: (Northwest and South West)

AFRICAN EGGPLANT DISHES

African eggplant soup (African garden eggs, meat, egusi, and other ingredients are used.), **African eggplant stew, Smoked pork aubergine soup, Garden egg sauce, African eggplant sauce, and Tunisian aubergines**

Efige zong: is a puree of the African eggplant fruit. It is a traditional dish of the Beti ethnic group of the South regions of Cameroon cooked in groundnuts.

Mendim me zong: is a delicacy highly appreciated by the Bulu ethnic group of the South region of Cameroon. It is a fruit juice served with boiled plantains to special guests to welcome them and express friendship. It is also consumed during lengthy discussion sessions or cases, and also given to women who have just given birth to cleanse the womb.

African eggplant in yellow soup: is a traditional dish from the Northwest region particularly Bafut in Mezam Division who use the dried eggplant to thicken the Achu soup. The Bamilike used the fresh one in their soup.

Aubergine au gratin: it is a low- fat dish.

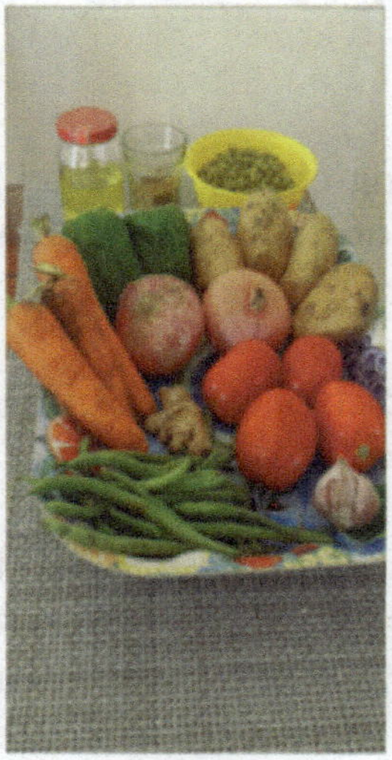

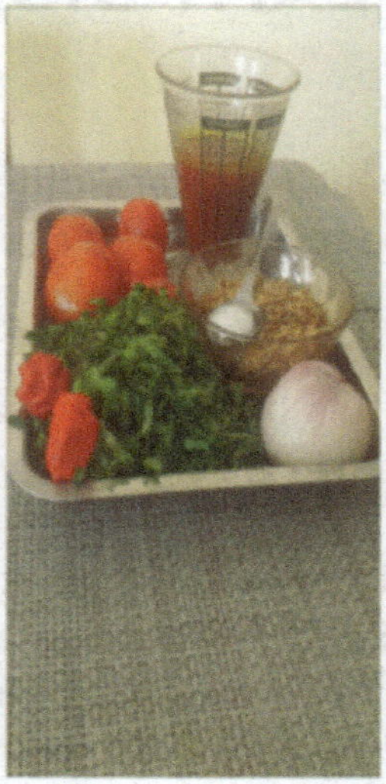

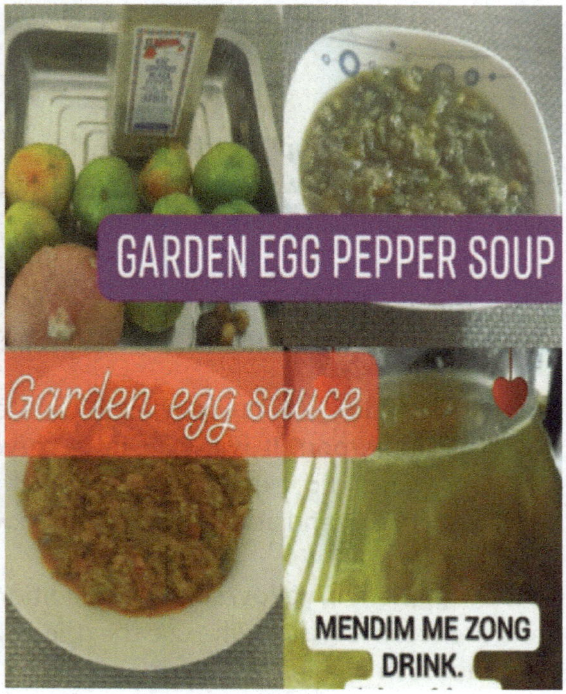
GARDEN EGG PEPPER SOUP
Garden egg sauce
MENDIM ME ZONG
DRINK.

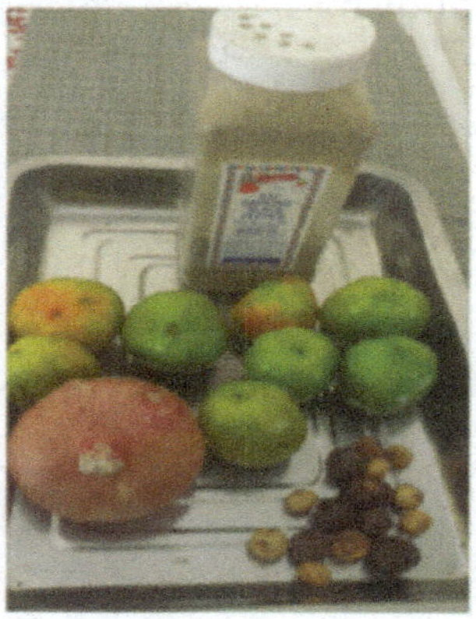

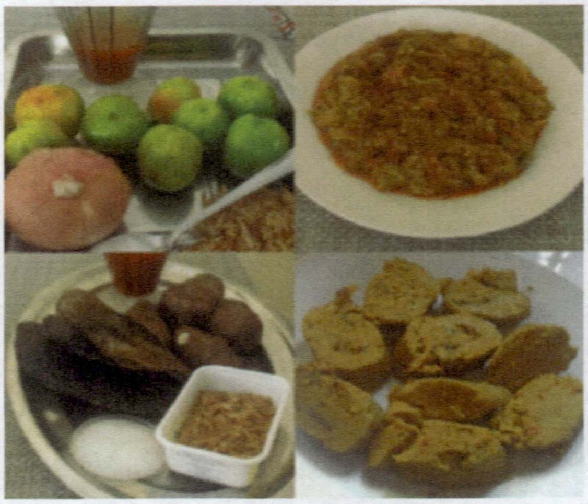

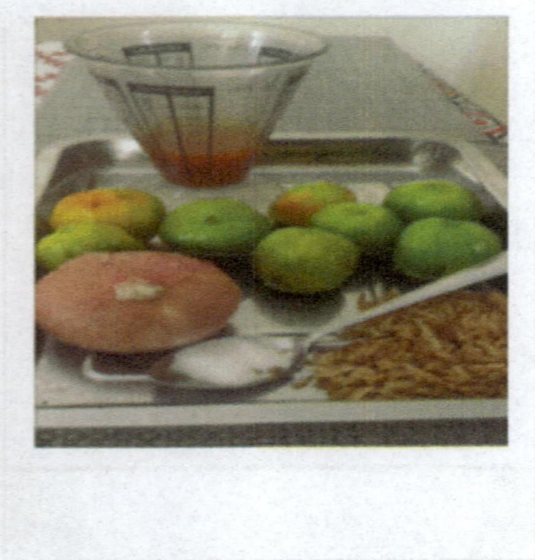

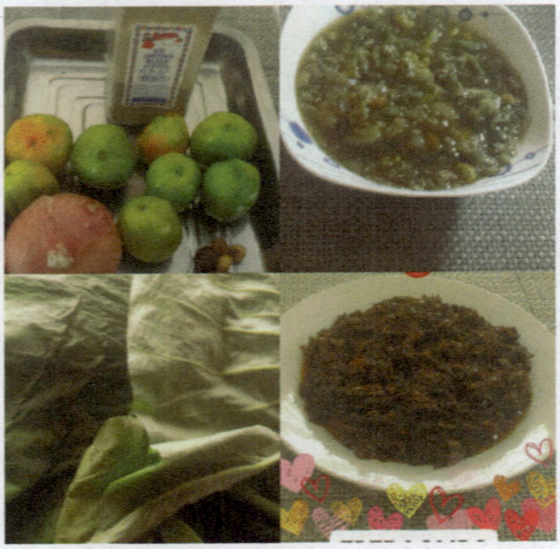

THE ERU LEAF

The eru leaf is a hard leaf from a leguminous plant. The botanical name for this plant is Gnetum spp. The leaves of the Gnetum spp are eaten throughout the Republic of Cameroon and have very many local names. The eru leaves are used to cook soup for the carbohydrate's staple foods of Cameroon.

The name "Eru" is from the Bayang people of Many Division of the South West Region of Cameroon. In the Centre and South Regions of Cameroon it is known by the following names okok by the Bakaka and Beti people, ikok by the Bassa people, ikiokio by the Yambassa people, and kiwa by the Bafia people. In the East Region the Bissom and the people of Yokadouma called it koko, while the Douala people of the Littoral Region call it ekoke. The Bankon people call it kóge. The neighboring Republic of Congo called it fumbua.

Since it is a hard forest leaf, it is softened in cooking by some other vegetables and ingredients. As a prominent soup of the people of Manyu Division of the South West Region, they use waterleaf of the spinach family to soften the eru leaf. The Beti people cook theirs in palm nut jus called nsougi, and with lots of groundnuts. The Yambassa and Bafia people of the Centre Region cook it also in palm nut jus, with either egusi or groundnuts, while the pigmies' slice koko thinly and cook in oil.

ERU DISHES

Eru soup: Bayang style is the eru soup cooked by the people of Manyu Division of the South West Region of Cameroon. Wild spinach or water leaf or young colocasia leaves are used to soften the hard eru leaves. Egusi is used in this soup.

Eru: is the most frequently used method in the preparation of eru in the North West and South West Regions. No thickening agent is used.

Okok: is cooked by the Beti and Bakaka people. They cook it with groundnuts and can be cooked also with soya bean powder.

Ikok: is cooked by the Bassa people. They use roast groundnut paste and egusi paste in palm nut jus called nsougi.

GLUTINOUS PRODUCTS AND SOUPS

A. OKRO (OKRA)

SCIENTIFIC NAMES: Abelmoschus callei, Abelmoschus esculentus,

COMMON NAMES: okro or okra

LOCAL NAMES: Pés (Eton), Bascodé (Fulfudé), Bitétam (Bulu, Ewondo), Koye (Bassa), Akro (Bamileke), Kigang (Douala), Gbarack à budum (Bafia), Koubeawa (Hausa), Ha (Bamoun), Akagang (Ngemba)

B. JUTE MALLOW

SCIENTIFIC NAMES: Corchonis olitonrius L, C tridens L, C trilocularis

COMMON NAME: Jute mallow

LOCAL NAMES: Tegue (Bulu, Ewondo), Lalo (Fulfulde, Hausa), Gbarack (Bafia) Nkelang (Bamileke), Teuere Messi (Bamoum), Keleng keleng (Douala), Django (Bassa), Cren cren (North West and South West Regions

C. AFRICAN MANGO

SCIENTIFIC NAME: Irvingia gabonensis

COMMON NAME: Wild Mango

LOCAL NAMES: Ndotuah, mpiang nouak (Eastern Region) agbono, dika nuts (Nigeria), Njanka, Manguis (Sanbage)

D. NKWI (NKWORO): Hibiscus-like stems

GLUTINOUS SOUPS

OKRO SOUP: It is cooked with mixed meat, smoked fish and okro with other ingredients.

OKRO SOUP, GHANANIAN VERSION: It is okro cooked with garden eggs, eggplant in oil.

THIN OKRO SOUP: is West African version of okro soup cooked with smoked meat or fish and fresh beef and other ingredients.

MIXED MEAT OKRO SOUP: It is a West African heavy okro soup with a variety of meats.

NKWORO SOUP: It is a Ngemba version of the Bamileke nkwi using the drawy stems of a shrub resembling hibiscus.

OKPOROKO AND AGBONO SOUP: It is a Nigerian soup of stock fish, beef, "ogwono" usually called bush mango and other ingredients.

OKRO SOUP: It is the Bamileke soup of okro, jute leaves called keleng keleng, thickened with ground nut paste.

NKWI: It is a special Bamileke soup of the stems of a plant of the hibiscus family with about ten indigenous medicinal spices incorporated in the soup.

CASSAVA LEAF SOUP: It is cassava leaves cooked with okro fruit, smoked fish and roast groundnut paste.

SOYA BEANS JUTE MALLOW LEAF SOUP: It is the jute leaves or keleng keleng or cren-cren cooked with beef and soya bean powder.

MPIANG NOUAK IS SOUP: of the East Region inhabitants in which the bush mango commonly called in the East as ndo chocolate is cooked with beef, and other ingredients.

BEEF OKRO SOUP: It is simple okro soup cooked with beef and other soup seasonings.

SAUCE DE LALO AU SOJA: It is soup of the inhabitants of North Cameroon soup with keleng-keleng (cren-cren) leaves cooked with beef and enriched with soya bean powder.

ASSOK BITETAM: It is an okro cake which is a traditional delicacy of the Beti community.

CHI NA'A: It is a traditional Bamileke yellow soup with okro.

GBARAK A TIEN: It is a Bamoun traditional dish of okro leaves and egusi.

EGUSI DISHES

Mukon ma ngondo: Is an elaborate egusi koki of pork and smoked fish of Bakweri people of the South West Region.

Nfian ngon: Beti style of egusi soup.

Kono ngon (ngonda'a mukon): Egusi koki with as its base.

Beef egusi soup: Soup cooked with beef, egusi, and okro.

Smoked chicken egusi soup: Egusi soup cooked with smoked chicken and egusi powder.

Egusi soup: Soup in which okro and cabbage is added.

Egusi koki: West African version of egusi pudding.

Nnam Nnam ngon: Beti style of egusi paste and smoked fish steamed in plantain leaves.

Sauce pistaches a la viande de boeuf: is a variety of egusi soup with okro.

Nfiang ndo'o: Egusi soup with ogwono.

MEAT

The Cameroonian soups are cooked with meat, beef being the most widely used. A pot of soup without meat included is a sign of poverty. The beef can be fresh or smoked. The skin of the cattle is eaten, usually called, “kanda” or “katanga.” It is considered meat for the poor but nowadays there are some soups that cannot be complete without the kanda. An occasion is considered grand in terms of how much meat is used, which means slaughtering one or more cows, goats, chickens etc.

Pork and goat meat is considered a delicacy and thus, not eaten daily at home. Pigs and goats are usually slaughtered by families during special occasions such as weddings, funerals, family get together, and other social gatherings. Mutton is not commonly eaten in daily meals. The intensity of its usage is when the Muslims celebrate their feasts, such as Feast of the Ram. It is then that the consumption of mutton is at its peak.

Nevertheless, in big cities there are special butcheries that sell all genres of meat. One can also find them in grocery stores, but which are very expensive, and unaffordable for the average Cameroonian.

Grilled goat, pork, sheep, fish and chicken are found at strategic street corners in the main cities. Together with ripe roast plantains, they offer lunch and dinner for a majority of people. Beef is also grilled, and it is called “soya.” There is goat soya and beef soya available at the entrance of bars and wherever people gather throughout the nation. There is a beef specialty in Cameroon which is called “kilichi.” It is spiced beef, sun dried, and grilled. It is crispy, tasty and can be preserved for months.

Cameroonians are great lovers of wildlife or game, usually called “bush meat.” It is cooked in soups, stewed, or steamed and can be used fresh or smoked. It is a delicacy which is scarce, and its hunting is controlled by government regulations so as to avoid the extinction of endangered species. Multiplied Daily allowances of meat are:

Infants and children need 10g per day multiplied by the age. E.g., A child of 6 years need 60g of meat per day, a 15-year-old need 150g per day.

Adults need 100g without bones per day, Manual workers need 150-200g per day, pregnant and lactating mothers need 150g per day. The elderly need 60-80g per day.

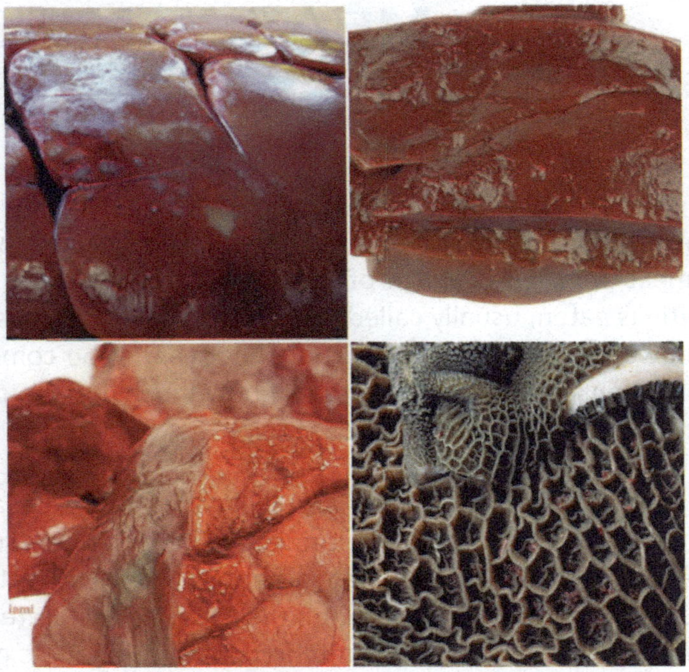

Kidneys, liver, lungs (fup-fup), tripe (towel)

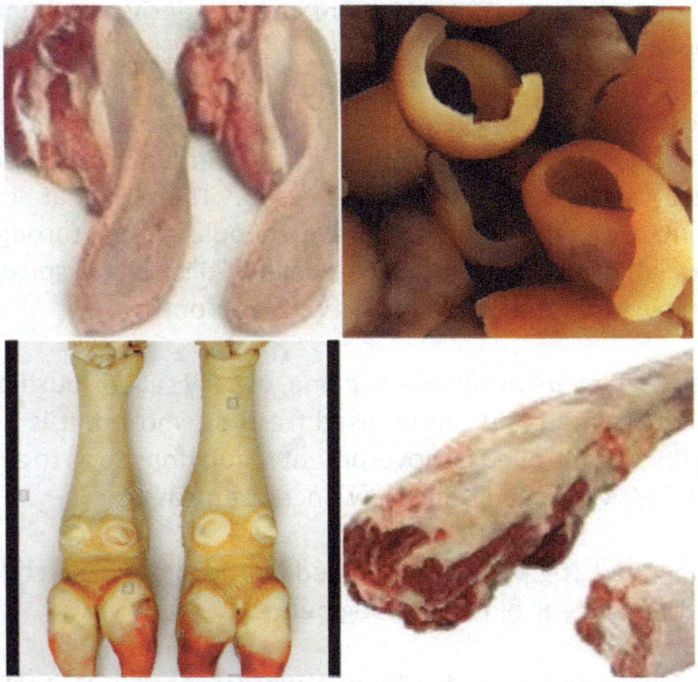

Tongue skin (kanda, katanga), foot cow, tail cow.

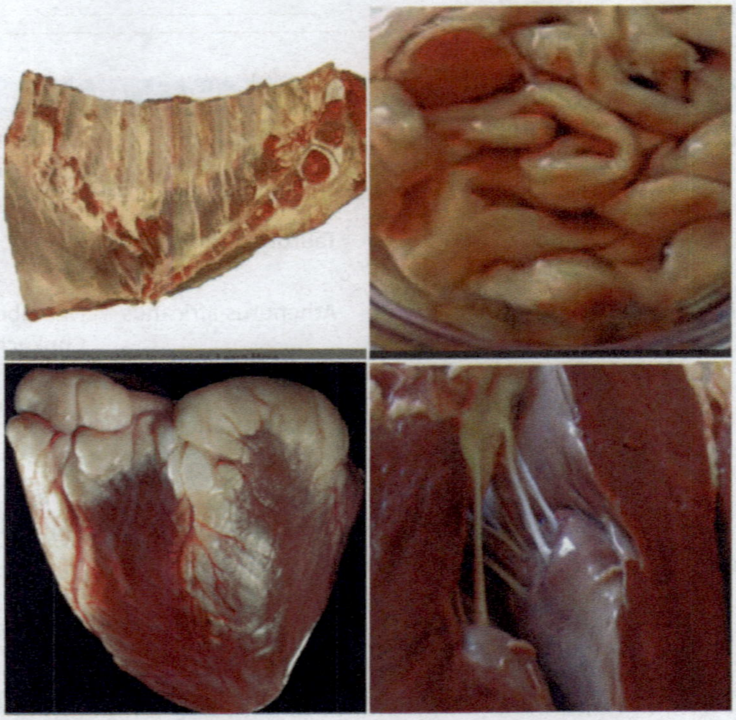

Brisket(biscuit bone), intestines (belle cow), heart cow.(full, cut)

SN	English name	French name	Scientific name	Common name
1.	Cattle (cow, bull)	Bétail (vache, caureau)	Bos indicus Bos brachyceros	Naagel (Fulbe) Nyaaka (Bakweri)
2.	Goat	Chèvre	Capra hircus	Mboli Mbee (Ngemba)
3.	Pig	Porc	Sus scrofa	Kwunyam (Bafut) Kfunyam (Ngemba) Ngoa
4.	Sheep (Ram, lamb)	Mouton	Ovis sp	Bélier, agneau, mulengu

GAME "BUSH MEAT"

SN	English name	French name	Scientific name	Common name
1.	African civit cat	Civitte d'Afrique	Civittictis civitta	Bush cat Jambo, chat Samvage
2.	Antelope	Antilope	Taurotragus oryx	Kavé Eland
3.	Brushed-tailed porcupine	Porc-épic	Athenurus africanus	Ngombe Chukuchuku beef
4.	African bush cat	Chat	Felis domestica	Eso
5.	Buffalo	Buffle	Syncerus caffer	Bush cow Njika
6.	Bush dog	Chien	Speothos Venaticus	Njue Vinegar dog Water dog
7.	Red river hog	Sanglier	Potamocherus Larvatus	Ngoa Wanga Bush pig
8.	Cane rat	Agouti	Thryonomys Swinderianjs	Merissan Cutting grass
9.	Deer	Chevreuil Daim	Cervus sp	Mbalu Kave
10.	Elephant	Eléphant	Loxodonta (Africana)	Njoku
11.	Giant rat	Rat de champs géat	Cricetomy gambianus	Poached rat
12.	Hare	Lièvre	Lepus camiculus	
13.	Putty-nosed monkey	Singe	Cercopithecus nicititans	Monkey

MEAT DISHES

1. **Soya** is open fire roast meat, be it goat, beef, chicken, mutton, or pork.
2. **Meat balls:** Steak, ground beef, sausage meat is used in meat balls.
3. **Bird's nest** is ground meat shaped into rings, have eggs broken into the rings and fried.
4. **Pepper liver** is marinated liver fried in oil and mixed with chives and green peppers.
5. **Braised steak** is steak pan braised in flour coating.
6. **Beef/ rice casserole** is rice cooked with courgette.
7. **Kilichi** is dried, grilled, and well-seasoned strips of meat.
8. **Beef/ potato** curry is a type of pottage.
9. **Onion Livers** is calf liver cooked in onions.
10. **Jamaican casserole** is when meat is rolled in seasoned flour and cooked in tomatoes.
11. **Flemish beef stew** is beef rolled in flour and the liquid used is beer.
12. **Goulash is beef stew** with Irish potatoes.
13. **Czech goulash** is beef stew thickened with flour.
14. **Mona style beef cabbage** is beef cooked in cabbage and courgette.
15. **Beef curry** is Lesotho style of curry stew.
16. **Delicious tomato stew.**
17. **Beef soya** is West African version of charcoal grill beef.
18. **Dijon kidney** is kidney cooked in French mustard.
19. **Tomato stew.**
20. **Foot cow (calf trotters) pepper soup is a Cameroonian delicacy**
21. **Tripe and onions** is tripe cooked in milk.

PROTEIN DELICACIES

There are some scarce delicacies in the Cameroonian cuisine such as snails, caterpillars, palm grubs or palm weevils, termites, grasshoppers, and crickets. They are eaten fresh, or dried and sautéed in spices and oil. They are seasonal, except for snails, which are not cultivated in large quantities, thus cannot feed a reasonable population

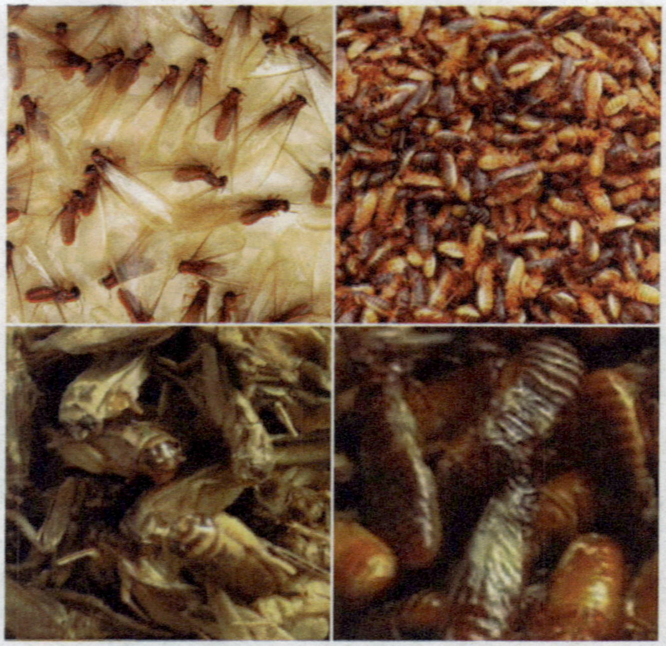

Raw termites, fried termites (ngoh), raw crickets, fried crickets

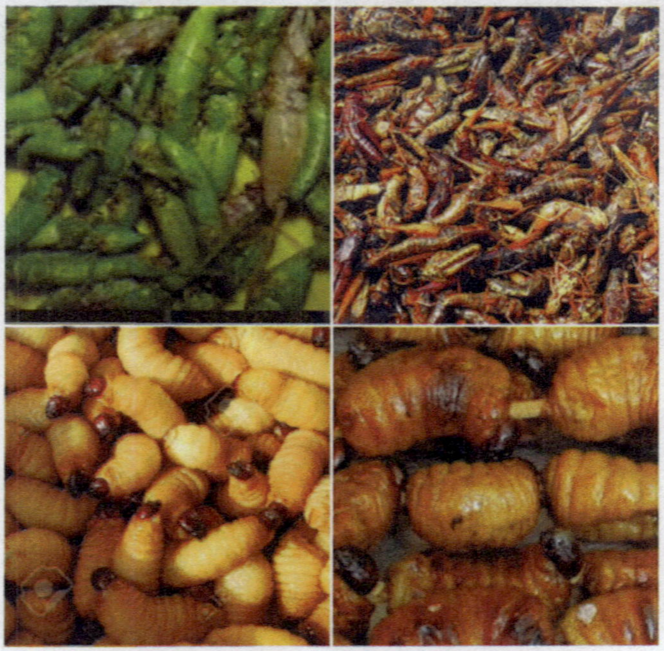

Fresh green grasshoppers, fried green grasshoppers (mungwin), fresh palm grubs/worms, fried palm grubs.

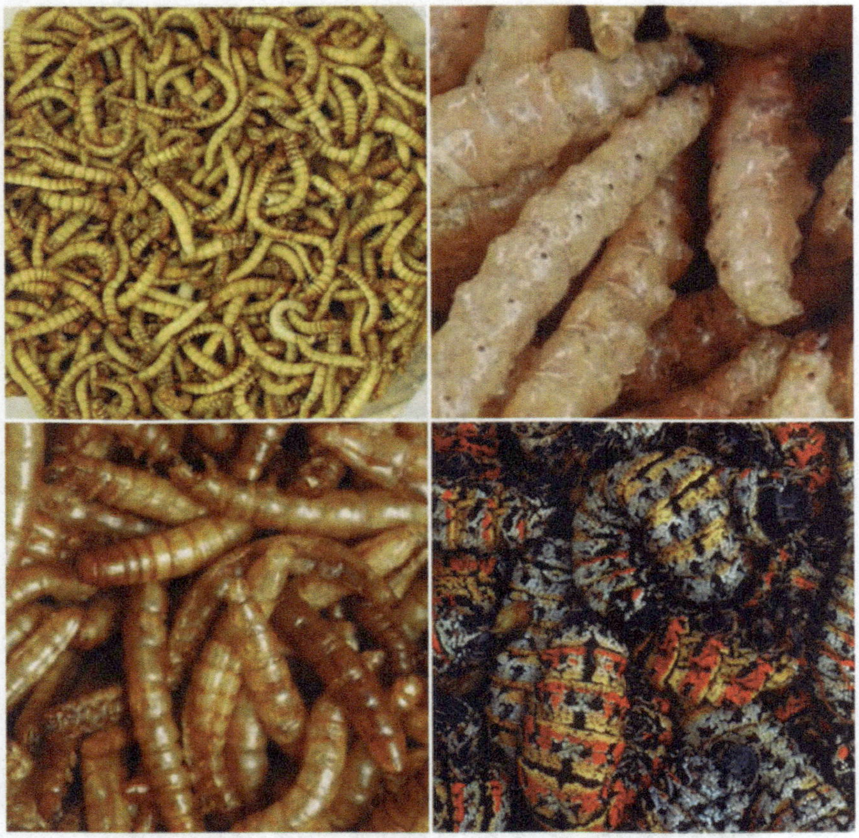

Edible caterpillars (worms/larvae)

KILICHI

Kilichi is meat, generally beef, which is dried, grilled in strips, and spiced with spices pastes. It is a traditional product of North Cameroon, a zone that produces a lot of beef. This dried meat is generally eaten as a crinkled product. If kilichi is well dried it can be preserved for more than six months. It is a highly prized product and can be exported but the quality is very irregular. The drying and grilling improves the dehydration of the meat in order to have a longer preservation period. A well prepared kilichi can last for long only if it is kept away from moisture and water. Beef is dried, spiced and grilled according to traditional processes by butchers.

The processes are as follows:

CLEANING: The parts of beef chosen for kilichi are the sirloin (tenderloin) and the thighs because they are attractive. Once these parts are selected, they are cleaned of their fat and cut into strips or chopped with the help of a small machete or a kitchen knife.

FIRST STAGE OF DRYING: The beef strips are placed on a shelf or screen and placed in the sun for 4-5 hours. It is turned often so that all the sides receive the sun. In order to avoid dust on the meat, drying is generally on the screen side well managed so that the dust is on the slab for example.

SPICING: The meat strips are spiced by soaking or marinating in a sauce of ground groundnuts, salt, onions, and other traditional spices. The quantity of spices used depends on the quantity of the meat to be dried. In this case one obtains reddish kilichi if soaked in spicy sauce with pepper and yellowish with spicy sauce without pepper.

SECOND STAGE OF DRYING: The meat strips are put to dry for 2 - 3 hours. It is steeped in oil and placed on a grill where it is carefully smoked over the heat fire. The duration of drying on the grill depends on the quality of the kilichi which can vary between 4-5 days for the quantities destined for commercial purposes.

A product very well appreciated and consumed by the population is obtained. Large quantities of the meat can be preserved and stocked for a long period. Most often kilichi is eaten in the crinkled state but it can be used in salads. The appearance of the product (color, look, flavor) and the chewing state (crispiness, toughness) are the criteria which the populations use to appreciate the quality of kilichi.

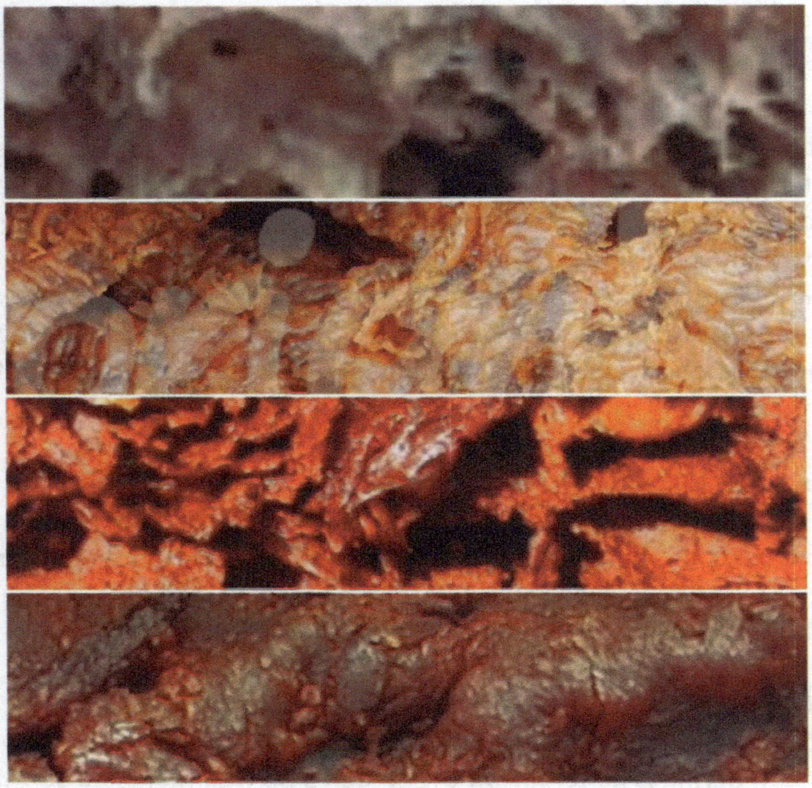

Kilichi (dried/smoked beef)

POULTRY AND POULTRY PRODUCTS

Among poultry products, Cameroon cuisine is uses mostly chicken and eggs. Ducks are available but are eaten by a few. Chickens are locally bred, whereas there are large poultry farms belonging to individuals and to companies. Partridges often called tsoh or bush fowl is usually got from hunters who bring their catch in very small quantities.

Ducks are usually called duck fowls. There are no large breeding houses for ducks. Sometimes some wings and drumsticks are found in cold stores. Turkeys are a scarce poultry product also.

Eggs are eaten hard boiled and hawkers sell them. They are eaten with pepper sauces. There are some hawkers who prepare fast sandwiches using boiled eggs. There are roadside small restaurants known as café houses. Throughout the day fast foods are prepared using omelets, spaghetti, and bread.

Local hens are reared by villagers in the country known as "country fowls" are tastier and firmer than those fed artificially

SN	ENGLISH NAME	FRENCH NAME	SCIENTIFIC NAME	COMMON NAMES
1.	Chicken	Poulet	Gallus domesticus	Uva Ngoub (Ngemba)
2.	Duck	Canard	Anas sp	Elela Duck fowl
3.	Partridge	Pintade	Numida meleagris	Bush fowl Kpaee Guinéa fowl Tsoh
4.	Pigeon	Pigeon	Columba sp	
5.	Egg	Oeuf	-	Meco

CHICKEN DISHES

Chicken and plantain DG, chicken CEO: Chicken DG is chicken cooked in plantains and a variety of vegetables.

Chicken fricassee: is chicken coated with flour and browned. Moisten with white wine.

Grilled chicken: Cameroon style is chicken marinated and oven grilled.

Keshk sauce: It is an Egyptian soup cooked with chicken breast in yogurt and flour.

Basque chicken: It is chicken cooked in white wine.

Khatii-khatii: It is a specialty of the people of Kom in the North West Region of Cameroon. It is chicken chopped and mixed with palm oil.

Chicken Dijon: It is chicken cooked with Dijon mustard.

Fresh herb grilled chicken: It is marinated chicken for 6 hours and roasted on a grill.

Poulet du capitaine.

Blanc de poulet à Provençale.

Le pepe soupe de poulet.

Zalam-zalaina: It is chicken pepper soup of the Massa people of North Cameroon and South Chad.

DG OR LE POULET DG

Le poulet DG is a Cameroonian dish of a fricassee of chicken, vegetables, and savory dishes. The name DG means Directeur Générale which in English means General Manager or Chief Executive Officer. When translated this dish will mean CHICKEN CEO i.e., Chicken Executive Officer.

This signifies that this dish was for the upper class, or for very important people. It was popular in the 1980's to meet the tastes of CEO's who wanted to eat full meals quickly away from home. For this dish to be served to important guests, the chicken itself had to be of the best quality, thus a GM itself.

The green, red, and yellow peppers simulate the colors of the Cameroon flag. The poulet DG's were served at small tables d'hote or "chantiers." These were not formal restaurants. They were called "chicken parlors. Chantiers or chicken parlors by Cameroonians were run by Cameroonian ladies who looked forward to making extra cash.

EGG DISHES

Scotch egg: This is also called birds' nests are scotch eggs prepared with sausage meat.

Egg ratatouille: It is egg fried and put on the ratatouille.

Oeuf en tomate: It is stuffed tomatoes with eggs and baked.

Sardine Omelet.

SEAFOOD AND FISH

Cameroonians cook fish in various ways such as fried, grilled, braised, steamed, boiled, and stewed. Smoked fish is a special favorite because preservation of fresh fish is difficult. Mackerel is the most common fish eaten by most households. Mackerel and sardines are considered fish for the poor. Imported stock fish is a delicacy for the very rich, due to its expense. Lean fish is sole, stock fish, whiting, and hake fish. Semi-fatty fish is mackerel and herring. Fatty fish is eel and tuna.

FISH DISHES

Fresh fish stew: Fish is fried before it is used to prepare stew.

Fresh fish Irish stew: Onion and tomatoes are fried first, other ingredients are then added, and the fish is the last thing to add, which is not fried.

Fresh fish pepper soup: It is a typical Cameroonian soup with njangsa as a thickening agent and which adds flavor and oil, **Kribi fish sautéed in garlic, Braised prawns.**

Grilled fish marinated overnight. Grill over open coals or in the oven, **Grilled bar, or sole Cameroonian Style.**

Sole au jus d'orange: It is frying fish in very shallow fat.

Poisson à l'oseille et aux arachide: It is smoked fish cooked in sorrel (folere) leaves and groundnuts is a Dish of the North of Cameroon.

Poisson à l'oseille: A Fulbe dish consisting of cooking fresh fish and sorrel leaves.

Ebangeh: Fish, pepper, and lemon soup of the people of Kribi, The Grand Batanga.

Mbongo Chobi soup: Ebony back soup of the Bassa people.

MBONGO TCHOBI

The caviar of the Bassa people, of the Littoral region of Cameroon, is the mbongo tchobi. It is a typical Bassa dish, it is a tasty and aromatic soup made from spices typical of Cameroon. The mbongo (Aframomium citratum) is a wild pepper that resembles the nutmeg in structure. This is the principal spice that gives the soup it flavors. One other spice for this soup is the hiomi, which is the bark of the garlic tree, the Davida.

The preparation of the soup is very long and tedious. It is necessary to use a day for the burning and mixing of aromas and condiments that make up the soup. Tchobi is fish in the Bassa language, thus the name of the soup mbongo tchobi. This soup is also known simply as mbongo which is an earthly spicy black tomato-based sauce with a smooth, thick, and velvet structure. Its distinctive taste and color are achieved by burning of the hiomi (mbongo stick) back of the Davida tree over open flame. It is then blended and incorporated into the tomato stew with other spices such as the grains of paradise, and njangsa (African wood-oil seed), and pebe, the African nutmeg.

SN	ENGLISH NAME	FRENCH NAME	SCIENTIFIC NAME	COMMON NAME
1.	Barracuda	Barracouta or brochet	Sphyraena	Kuta, Muawu, barra, Pollock, haddock
2.	Cod Fish	Morue	Gadus morrhua	Stock Fish, Mukanjo
3.	Common whelk (snails)	Buccin	Buccinum undatum	Bulot
4.	Sea Bass	Daurade dorade	Sparus aurata	Orate (Italy) Dorada (Spain) Common dolphin fish
5.	Eel	Anguille	Anguilla Anguilla	Caviar Snake fish
6.	Land crab	Crabe de terre	Cardisoma guanhumi	Crab
7.	Herring	Hareng	Clupia harengs	Mbonga, Welolo
8.	Lobster	Langouste	Humarus vulgaris	
9.	Mackerel	Maquereau	Scomber sp	
10.	Mullet	Mulet	Mugil cephalus	Grey mullets, red mullets, Goat fish, surmullet
11.	Oyster	Huître	Ostrea sp	
12.	Sardine	Sardine		Sardine fish

13.	Salmon	Saumon	Salmo salar	Atlantic salmon, Bay salmon, black salmon
14.	Shine nose	Carpe, tanche	Chinook tshawytscha	Black mouth, King tyee, chino salmon
15.	Shrimps	Crevettes	Crangon vulgaris	Dibanga, écrevisse, crayfish, njanga, medjanga
16.	Skate	Raie	Raja anguilla	-
17.	Snails	Escargots	Gastropoda	Nyamngoro, Ataa (Ngemba)
18.	Sole	Sole	Solea solea	Dover sole
19.	Turtle	Tortue	Chelonia sp	
20.	Hog fish	Capitaine	Lachnolaimus maximus	Mbuta, nile perch, Lake Victoria perch, Nile fish,
21.	Tuna (yellow fin)	Thon	Thunnini	Bullet tuna
22.	Bonito	Bonite	Thunnini	Skipjack tuna
23.	Grouper	Mérue	Epinephelus mycteroperca	Sea basses groper (Australia) Hammour (Middle East)
24.	Tortoise	Tortue	Testudo sp	Ikulekule
25.	Catfish	Machoiron		Silurid, Mud fish
26.	Tilapia	Carpe		

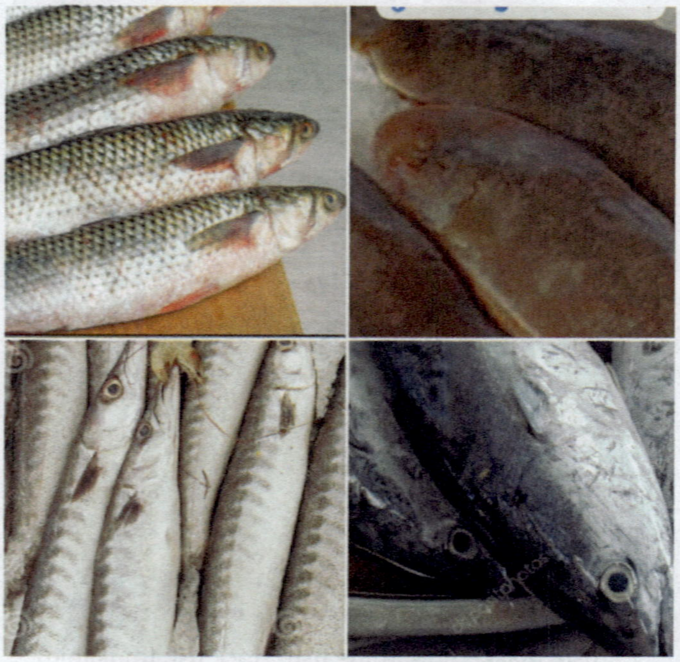

Mullet, sole, barracuda (kuta, brochet), tuna(tong)

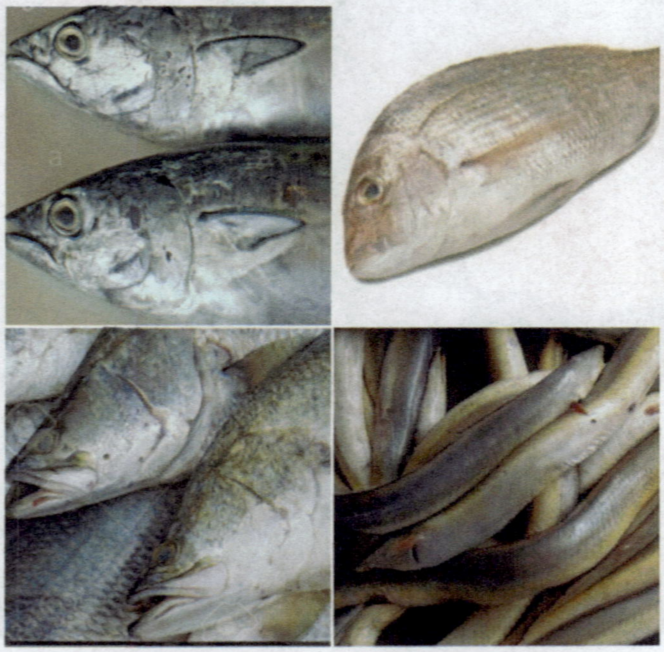

Bonito (bonite, shine nose (carpe), sea bass (dorade), eel (snake fish)

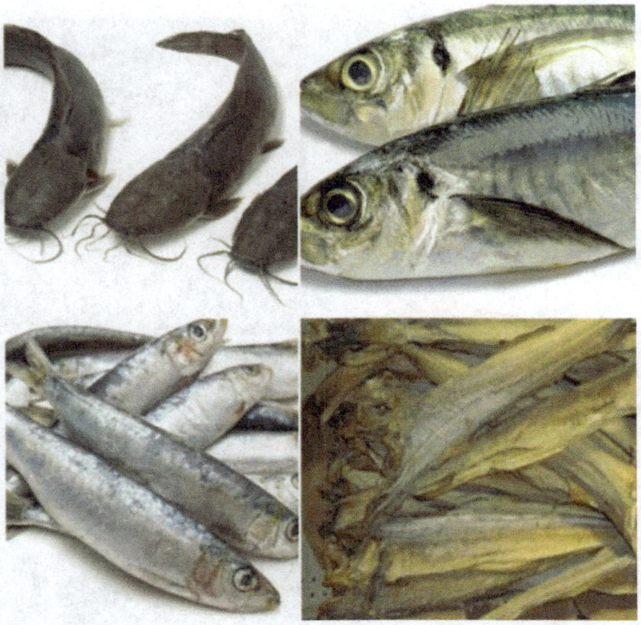

Catfish, mackerel, sardine fish, stock fish (mukanjo)

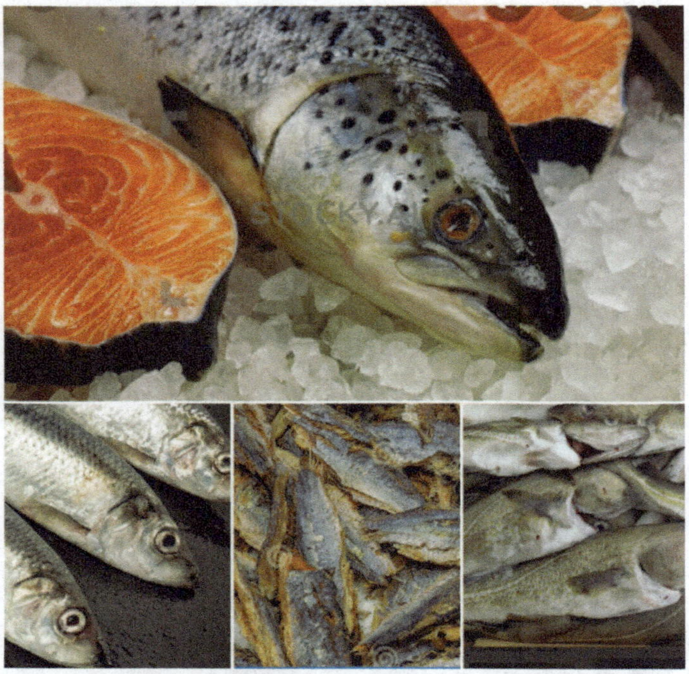

Salmon, fresh herring, dried herring (mbonga/strong kanda), cod fish

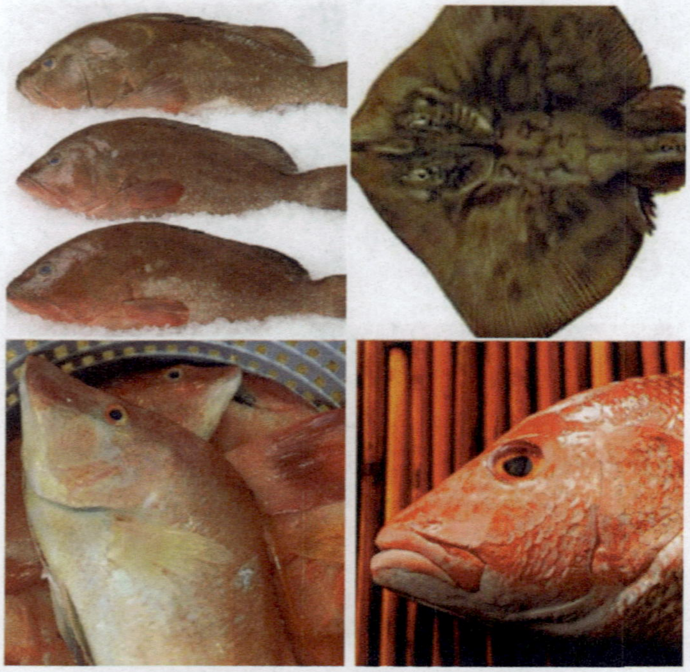

Grouper (sea bass), skate fish (cover pot), hogfish (capitaine), Snapper (capitaine)

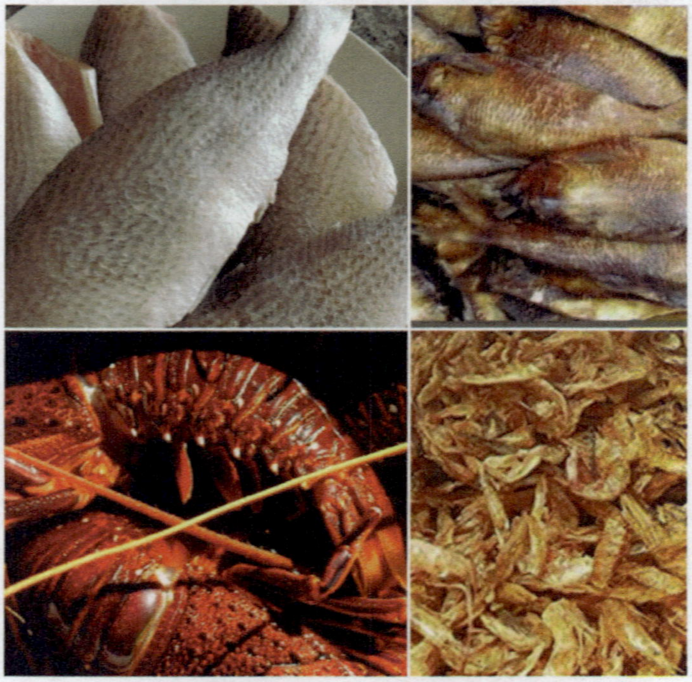

Croaker, herring (mbonga), lobster, crayfish (njanga)

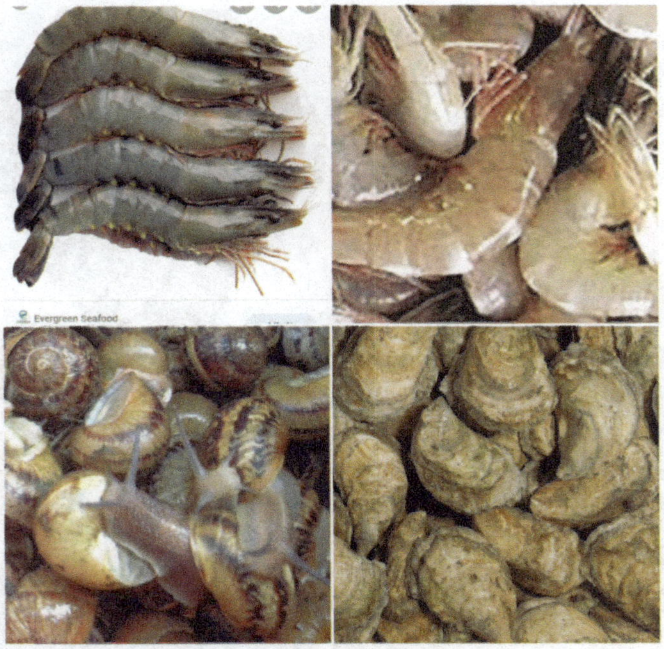

Prawns, shrimps, snails, oysters.

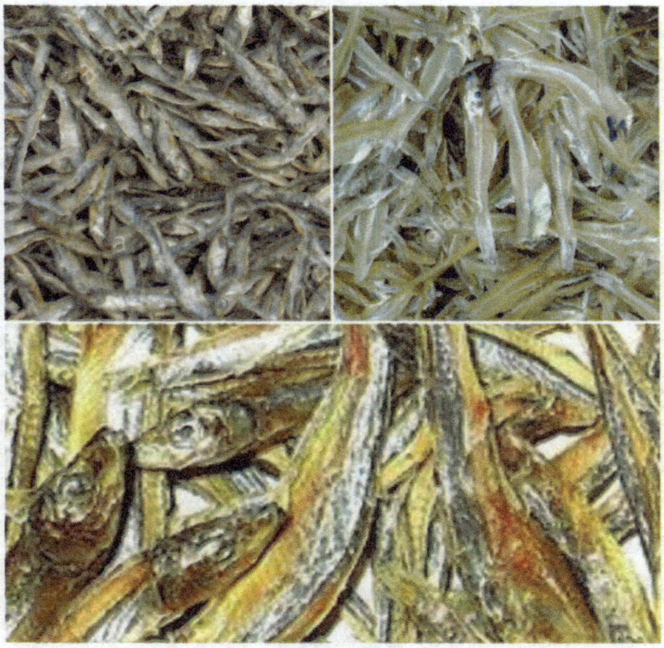

Anchovy (die no cover eye, milolo)

NDOMBA DISHES

Ndomba, domba, or Bomba are dishes typical of the Yaounde people. They are neither soups nor stews but are accompaniments to the starchy foods. They are steamed, grilled and are roasted in hot ashes. It uses many traditional spices.

Meat domba: It is a Yaounde traditional dish. Meat such as goat is used and spiced with herbs.

Fish ndomba: It is well seasoned fresh fish with native spices and herbs.

Bomba de volaille: It is spice chicken steamed in banana leaves or aluminum foil paper.

Domba de silure: It is soft water fish domba

Ndomba de porc au citron: It is pork ndomba spiced with many spices including lemon juice.

Chicken domba: It is chicken spiced with traditional spices, tied in plantain leaves, and steamed.

Mpub fish: It is the Bakossi version of fish ndomba coated with plantain flour.

Liphele: It is the Bakweri version of fish ndomba.

FRUITS

Cameroon is a haven for fruits such as Mangoes, plums, pineapples, oranges, grapefruits, lemons, limes, passion fruits, avocados, bananas, and pawpaws which are seasonal. When in season they are affordable to everyone. Some fruits such as apples and grapes, which are imported, are found in grocery stores or supermarkets in big cities and along the streets in the main cities. Cameroonians like sweet fruits and they snack on them throughout the day.

SN	ENGLISH NAME	FRENCH NAME	BOTANICAL NAME	COMMON NAME
1.	Apple	Pomme	Malus pumille (sylvestris)	
2.	Avocado	Avocat	Presea Americana	Pear, alligator pear Bia (Ngemba) Butter fruit, butter pear
3.	Banana	Banane	Musa Ocuminata	Amboe (Ngemba)
4.	Bread fruit	Fruit à pain	Artocarpus communis	Pfutu
5.	Grapefruit	Pamplemouse	Citrus paradise	Pomelo, molanjo
6.	Guava	Goyave	Psidium guajava	
7.	Guyabano	Corossol hérissé	Annona muriciata	Sour sop
8.	Lemon	Citron	Citrus limon	
9.	Lime	Limon, citron vert	Citrus aurantifolia	Njofinua
10.	Mango	Manguea	Mangifera indica	
11.	Mangosteen	Mangosta	Garcinia mangostana	Ntangnu (Ngemba)
12.	Plums	Plume	Dacryodes edulis	Butterfruit, bush butter obe, Ssa (Ewondo) safou, African pear, West African plum
13.	Pawpaw	Papaya	Carica papaya	Pfopfo
14.	Pineapple	Anana	Anana Comsus	Liange
15.	Sugar cane	Canne à sucre	Saccharum officinarum	Rechat (Fulbe) Mokoko Asisang (Ngemba)
16.	Orange	Orange	Citrus sinensis	
17.	Tangerine	Mandarine orange de tanger	Citrus reticulate	
18.	Watermelon	Pasteque	Citrullus vulgaris	Niboh
19.	Passion fruit	Fruit de passion	Passiflora edulis	Adam fruit Fruit d'Adam
20. 21.	Rambutan Monkey Kola		Cola Cola Caricifolia	

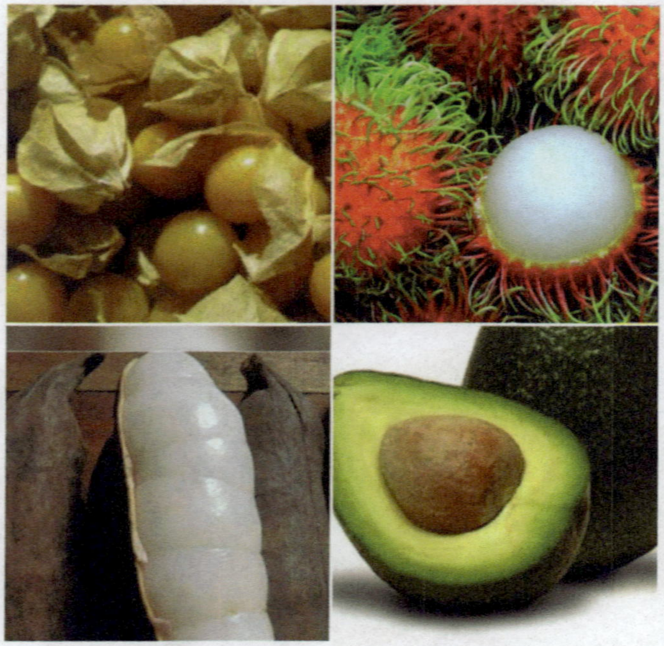

Ground berries, rambutan, monkey kola, pear (avocado)

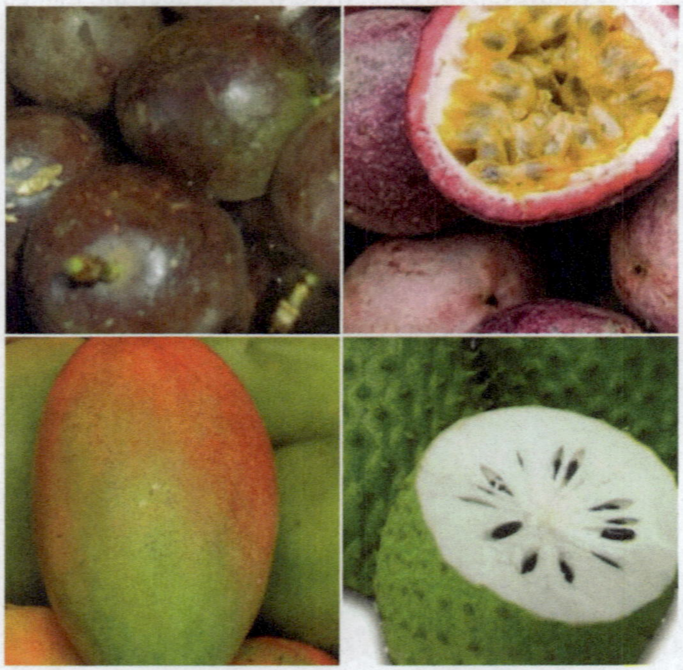

Adam fruit, passion fruit, mango, sour sop.

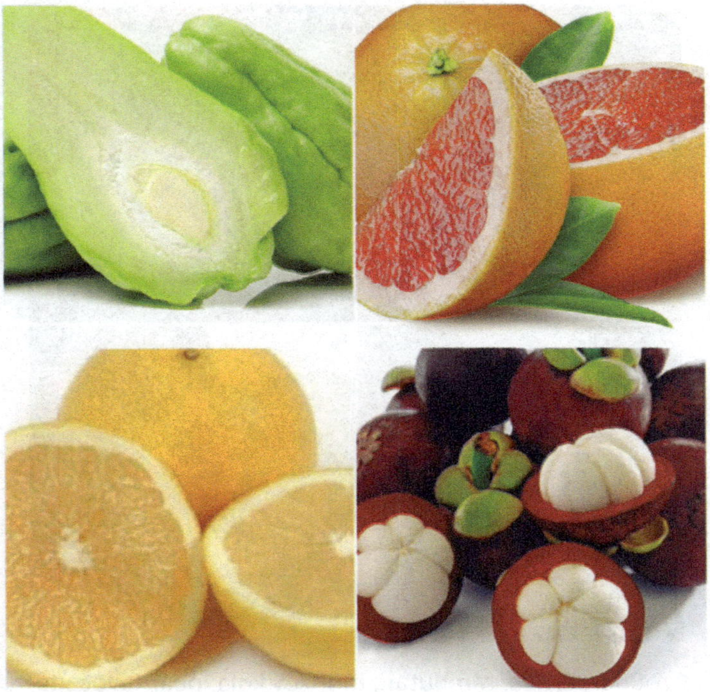

Christophines (chayote), red grapefruit, white grapefruit, mangosteen.

CAMEROON BUTTERY FRUITS

THE AFRICAN PLUM

A fruit with the botanical name Dacryodes edulis is what is commonly called in Cameroon as plum. Safou, African pear, African plum, Atanga in Gabon, butter fruit, nsafor bush butter, and bush pear are all names given to this fruit. It is a fruit with an odd flavor, a creamy buttery texture, a rich deep, oily pulp, pinkish when it is not ready and deep blue or violet whenit is ready to be harvested. It is a seasonal fruit harvested between the months of late May to late October.

The African plum is high in unsaturated fats, essential amino acids, proteins, vitamins, oil, and energy and low in salt. The plum is roasted in hot coals and ash, pot roasted by sprinkling with water or boiled in salted water in a very short time. When roasted or boiled in salted water, the pulp separates from the skin and seed and takes a buttery flavor. Too much high heat hardens it and renders it uneatable. Sometimes if exposed to the least heat it ripens and becomes soft and can be eaten without cooking, but the flavor is not appetizing. It can be eaten raw while still hard as colanuts, but the skin will not pull off of the seed, and there will be no pulp. The pulp is similar to that of the avocado in color.

The plum is usually eaten as a snack, alone or with roast or boiled corn and ripe or unripe roast plantains. It is a highly priced delicacy of Cameroonians, both young and old who wait anxiously for the harvesting season. There have not been any menus developed for the use of the African plum, but the menus of the avocado can use the plum as an alternative in place of the avocado.

THE AVOCADO

The pear is the name commonly used in Cameroon to refer to the avocado of the Persea americana family, which is a large berry containing a single seed. Alternate names to the avocado are alligator pear, butter pear, and aguacate. It is soft and slightly a flavored fruit.

It is high in calories, and fats (71-88%) but a source of pantothenic acid, dietary fiber, vitamin K, copper, folate, vitamin B6, potassium, and vitamins C and E. It is a seasonal fruit between the months of May and October and has many varieties.

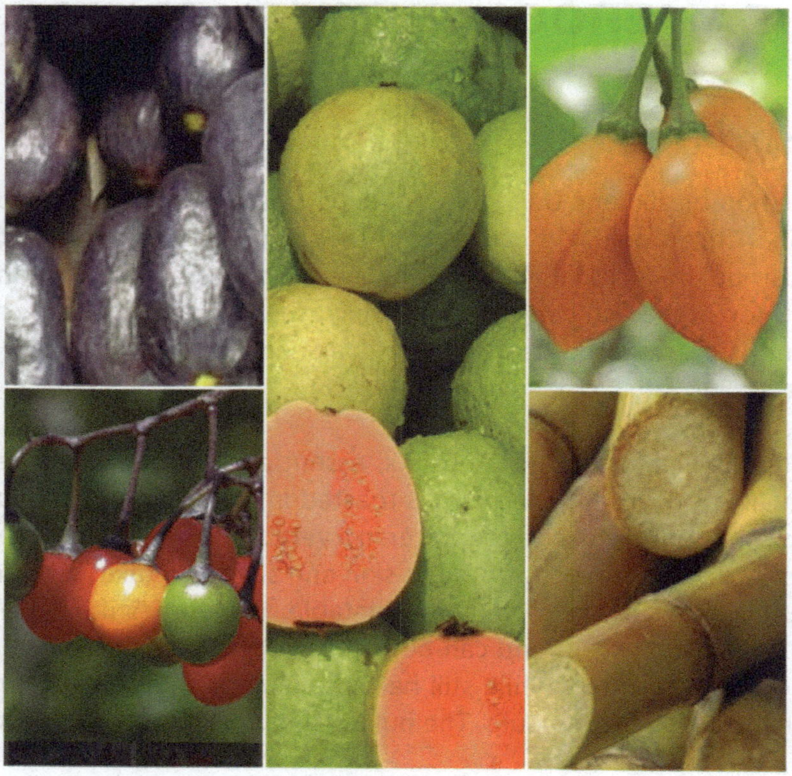

African plum, guava, tree tomato (night shade fruits), sugarcane.

NUTS AND BERRIES

Nuts are common in the Cameroonian diet as snacks. These nuts such as palm kernels, coconuts, cashew nuts, and groundnuts are common and affordable to everyone. The bitter kola and yellow kola are very bitter, used as stimulants, aids in digestion and used as items of socialization in occasions as death ceremonies, traditional wedding ceremonies or just any social occasion.

SN	ENGLISH NAME	FRENCH NAME	BOTANICAL NAME	COMMON NAME
1.	Bitter kola	Kola amère	Garcinia cola	Pulpe gorro (Fulbe) Nyaa-a (Ngemba)
2.	Kolanut	Noix de kola	Cola acuminate	Kolatier Pink cola Nibii (Ngemba)
3.	Cashew nut	Noix d'acajou (Anacardier)	Anacardium occidentale	Cashoi anacardier
4.	Coconut	Noix de coco (cocofia)	Cocos nucifera	Muangomo Likawe Cocofia Mbangkob (Bafut)
5.	Palmnut	Noix de palme	Elaeïs guineensis	Red mbanga Palmier Mbia Mbang (Bafut)
6.	Palm kernels	Amande de palmier	Elaeïs guineensis	Mbang Mbanga

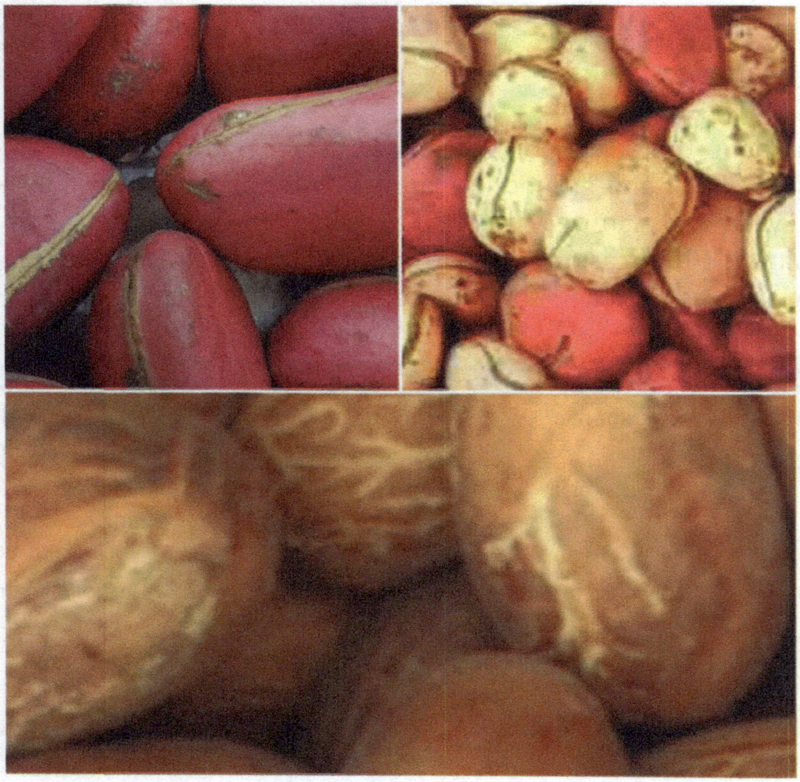

Colanuts, bitter colanuts.

PALM NUT JUS DISHES

Palm nut jus is a prized liquid used in cooking some Cameroonian dishes or soups. The fresh palm nuts are cooked in water, pounded in a mortar to obtain the jus or stock. It is washed and strained to recover the jus including oil. This liquid has many names such as mbanga soup which is cooked by the North West and South West people of Cameroon. The Beti people of the Centre Region call it Essouk while Sougi is the name given by the Bassa people of the same region and of Littoral Region.

PLAIN PALM NUT SOUP: It is a specialty of the South West Region of Cameroon.

PORCUPINE IN ESSOUK: It is porcupine cooked in mbanga soup by the Betis.

CHICKEN IN SOUGI: It is chicken cooked in mbanga soup by the Bassas.

ABENKWAIN: It is mbanga soup cooked in beef and okro by the Ghana people of West Africa.

NYONGA MOSAKA: It is palm nut soup of the Bakweri ethnic group.

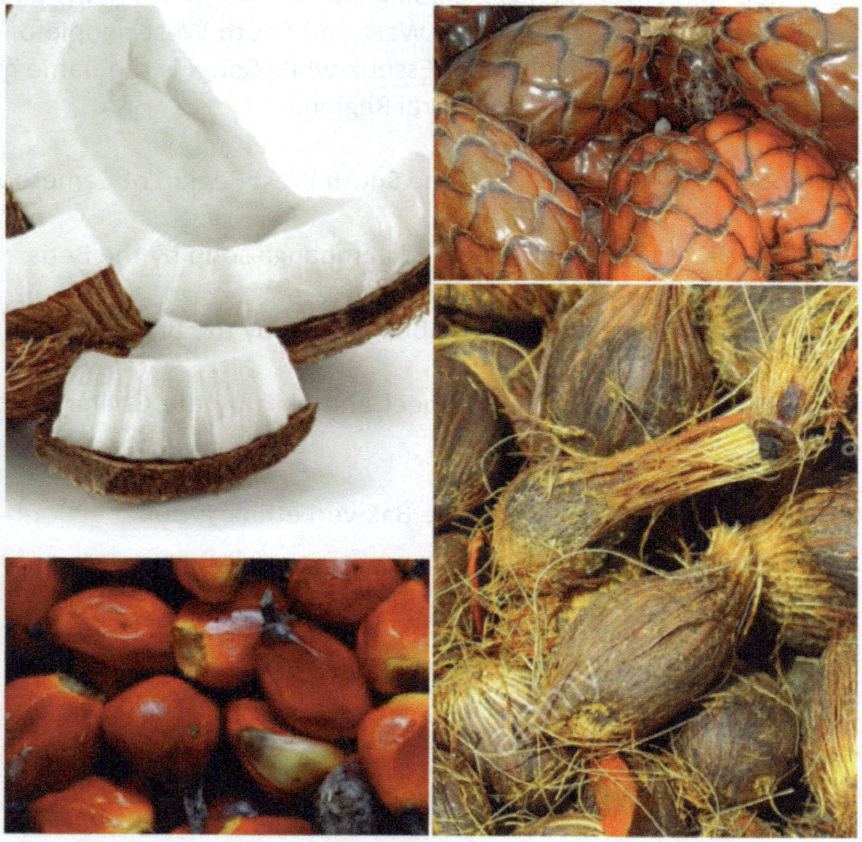

Coconuts, raffia palm fruit, palm nuts, palm kernels

PART TWO
MEAL AND MEAL PLANNING

A Meal is the food served and eaten at one sitting.

Meal planning is the programming of what you are going to serve for a certain amount of time. It could be a week, a day, or a month.

OBJECTIVES OF MEAL PLANNING

To make cheap meals, and save money, to make nutritious meals, and have a healthy family, to make a meal suitable for all of the family, to make meals in advance that can be frozen, to save time and effort, by reducing shopping time, Planning helps you make good use of leftovers. Planning helps to avoid shortages, spoilage, and poor feeding, to make balanced meals

TYPES OF MEALS

BARBECUE: It is a meal where food (often meat or fish) is cooked out of doors on an open fire or portable grill.

A BANQUET: It is a large formal, elaborate evening meal, with many guests followed by speeches in honor of someone.

A BUFFET: It is a meal whereby diners serve themselves from foods of several dishes placed in a public area. Buffets are good for serving large numbers of people at once as in institutional settings such as business conventions or large parties. Buffet is a French word meaning all you can consume.

PICNIC: A picnic is an outdoor meal where one brings one's food, such as a sandwich or a prepared meal (sometimes in a picnic basket). A picnic of ten takes place in a natural or recreational area, such as a park, forest, beach, or lawn, or a rest area on long drives at a roadside stop.

POTLUCK: It is a gathering of people where each person or group of people may contribute a dish of food prepared by the person or a group of people, to be shared among each group.

COCKTAIL PARTY (COCKTAIL RECEPTIONS): A party at which cocktails are served. When it is organized for purposes of social or business networking it is called a mixer. It is sometimes served between the hours of 4pm and 6pm. Some events, such as wedding receptions, are preceded by a cocktail hour. During the cocktail hour, guests socialize while drinking and eating appetizers.

MEALTIMES

The type of meal served or eaten at any given time varies by custom and location. In most cultures three meals are eaten, in the morning, early afternoon and evening. The names of meals are often interchangeable by custom. Breakfast is common to all cultures. In some cultures, region, or family the midday meal is called Lunch or Dinner and the evening meal supper. (Breakfast Lunch-Supper or Breakfast-Dinner-Supper)

BREAKFAST: It is eaten within an hour or two after a person wakes in the morning. Between 7:00 and 9:00a.m.

LUNCH: It is eaten around mid-day usually between 11am and 3pm or 12:00 and 1:30pm.

SUPPER OR DINNER OR TEA: It is eaten in the evening. Many English-speakers use "Supper" for this meal, 6:30pm and 8:00pm.

BRUNCH: This is a late-morning meal, usually larger than a breakfast and usually replacing both breakfast and lunch.

TEA: Refers to a meal in some commonwealth countries, such as Britain and Ireland. Teatime is the time at which the tea meal is usually eaten, which is late afternoon to early evening.

AFTERNOON TEA: It is a light meal typically eaten between 4pm and 6pm. Food is served on a tiered stand and it consists of bread, scones with butter or margarine, toast, muffins, or crumpets, maybe a glass of champagne or a similar alcoholic drink.

HIGH TEA (MEAT TEA): is one name for the evening meal between 5pm and 7pm in the UK. A hot dish, cakes, bread, butter, jam, cold cuts of meat e.g., ham salad are served.

BREAKFAST

Breakfast comprises of the following:

BEVERAGE

Tea, coffee, cocoa, Ovaltine, matinal, milk, lemon grass, water, etc.

CARBOHYDRATE DISH: Pap, Bread, Fried Plantains, Dodo), Fried Irish Potatoes

Cereal (Quaker oats, Corn Flakes, Puff-puff, Pasta)

PROTEIN: Eggs, Meat, Beans, and Bean products

FRUIT: Fruit juices, fruit drinks (mostly citrus fruits such as orange, lemon, grapefruit, lime)

BASIC TYPES OF BREAKFAST

These are types of breakfast served in hotels, in the hotel restaurant dining rooms or in the guest's bedroom or suites.

CONTINENTAL BREAKFAST OR CAFE COMPLET:

It is a light meal meant to satisfy a breakfaster until lunch. It originated from France. A typical continental breakfast consists of the following:

Juice	Mango juice, pineapple juice, tomato juice, orange juice, or grapefruit juice
Bread	Toast (white bread/brown bread), rolls, croissant, brioche, muffins, dough nuts, Danish pastry served with preserves, jam, honey, marmalade, and butter
Beverage	Hot beverage such as tea or coffee

The continental breakfast may also include sliced cold meats, such as salami or ham, and yogurt or cereal. Some countries of Europe, such as the Netherlands and those in Scandinavia, add a bit of fruit and cheese to the breakfast menu, occasionally even a boiled egg or a little salami.

If **tea** is served with the above breakfast, then it is known as "**The Complet**"

If **coffee** is served with the above breakfast, then it is known as "**cafe complet**"

If coffee alone is taken with nothing to eat, it is known as "**cafe simple**"

If the guest takes tea alone then it is known as "**The simple**"

The current trend in the continental breakfast menu includes a wide variety of choice of food items as follows:

Juice	**Mango, pineapple, orange, fresh apple, stewed fruit, strawberries, melon, tomato juice, grapefruit, (half or segments), figs, prunes (fresh and stewed.)**
Cereals	**Corn Flakes, Rice Crispies, Bran Flakes, porridge**
Yogurts	**Natural or fruit, regular or low fat**
Fish	**Grilled herring, fried or grilled sole, smoked fish, marinated fish**
Eggs	**Fried, poached, scrambled, boiled, plain or savory, filled omelet, eggs Benedict.**
Meats	**Bacon in various styles, various sausages, kidney, steak, gammon.**

Potatoes and vegetables	**Hash browns sauté potatoes, home fries, mushrooms, baked beans, fresh or grilled tomatoes.**
Pan cakes and waffles	**Regular pancakes or waffles with maple syrup or other toppings, blueberry pancakes, whole meal pancakes griddles cakes.**
Cold buffet	**Hams, tongue, chicken, smoked cold meats, salami, cheeses.**
Bread items	**Toast, rolls, croissants, brioches, crisp breads, plain sliced white or brown bread, Danish pastries.** **American muffins, English muffins, spiced scones, tea cakes, doughnuts**
Preserves	**Jams, marmalade, honey**
Beverages	**Tea, coffee, (including de caffeinated), chocolate, milk, mineral water**

ENGLISH BREAKFAST

An English breakfast is an elaborate breakfast quite substantial in size and variety. It is also called full breakfast or traditional breakfast. This traditional English breakfast comprises ten courses as follows:

Juice	**Chilled fruit juices pineapple, orange, apple grapefruit, tomato**
Stewed fruits	Apples, prunes, figs, pears etc. are cut into small pieces and cooked in sugar syrup flavored with clove and cinnamon. It is served in a cocktail cup with a quarter plate as under liner and the cutlery provided is a teaspoon.
Cereals	Oatmeal (meal), Corn Flakes, Wheat Flakes, Rice Crispies, and porridge served with cold or hot milk in a soup bowl with a quarter plate as under liner and a dessert spoon is provided as cutlery.
Fish	Herring, haddock, sardines are served
Eggs	Boiled, fried, poached, scrambled, plain or savory omelet
Meats	Fried or grilled bacon, sausages, ham, salami, kidney, or liver.
Rolls and toast	Toast white or brown, rolls like croissant, muffins, brioche doughnuts, Danish pastry.
Butter and preserves	Butter, jam, jelly, marmalade, honey, maple, syrup.
Fruits	Fresh fruits like melon, pawpaw, mango, orange, grapefruit, pears.
Beverages	Tea, coffee, hot beverages like bournvita, horlicks, Ovaltine, cocoa, milo.

AMERICAN BREAKFAST

Traditional breakfasts in the United States and Canada derive from the full English breakfast and feature predominantly sweet or mild-flavored foods, mostly hot.

The American breakfast comprises the following courses:

Juice	Mango, pineapple, orange, grapefruit, tomato
Cereals	Oatmeal (meal), Corn Flakes, Wheat Flakes, Rice, Crispies, and porridge served with hot or cold milk.
Eggs	Boiled, fried, poached, scrambled, omelet served with bacon, ham, or sausages.
Breads	Toast white or brown, rolls, brioche, and croissants with preserves like jam, jelly marmalade and honey.
Beverages	Tea, coffee, hot beverages like bournvita, milo, horlicks, Ovaltine.

INDIAN BREAKFAST

An Indian breakfast varies from region to region and is mostly vegetarian.

Juice	Mango, pineapple, orange, grapes, tomato
Fruit salad	Fresh, seasonal fruit accompanied with yogurt or honey.
Sweet dishes	Basmati rice, sweet porridge, sweetened, milk, rava, kesari, jalebi, halwa.
Eggs	Boiled eggs, omelet, scrambled eggs or white or whole meat bread toast served with crumbled homemade paneer cheese and chopped spinach
Breads	Toast or plain white/brown breads, butter sandwiches.
Indian specialty breakfast items	Idlis, vadis, dosas and chepatis served with sambar and chutneys.
Beverages	Tea, coffee, hot beverages like bournvita, milo, horlicks, Ovaltine.

LUNCH AND DINNER

Lunch may include the following:

Carbohydrates

Protein

Vegetables: (cooked or raw as in salads)

Fruits: fruit drinks/fruit salads

Desserts: (sweets such as cakes, pies etc.)

MEAL COURSES

A meal course is a specific set of food items that are served together during a meal, all at the same time. A course may include multiple dishes or only one, and often includes items with some variety of flavors.

A full course dinner is a dinner consisting of multiple dishes, or courses. It can consist of three or four courses such as appetizers, fish course, entree, main course, and dessert. In formal dining, a full course dinner can consist of 5, 6, 8, 10, 12 or 16 courses. In these formal dining events, the courses are carefully planned to complement each other gastronomically, the courses are smaller and spread out over a long evening up to three, four or five hours as follows:

A ONE COURSE MEAL: It is the Main Course

A TWO COURSE MEAL: It is an Appetizer, can be a soup or salad and the Main Course

A THREE COURSE MEAL: It is an Appetizer (soup or salad), the Main Course and Dessert.

A FOUR COURSE MEAL: It is a Soup, a Salad, a Main Course, and a Dessert.

A FIVE COURSE MEAL: It is a Soup, a Fish, the Main Course, a Salad, and a Dessert

A SIX COURSE MEAL: It is Hors d'oeuvres/appetizer, Soup, Fish, Main Course, Salad, and Dessert.

Most English speakers, France and parts of Canada call the first course "Entrée" while the USA and parts of Canada take it to mean the main course.

FIRST COURSE MEAL

A first course dish can be any of the following:

APPETIZER: An appetizer is a small dish of food or drink taken before a meal or the main course of a meal to stimulate one's appetite. This is the first course of a meal.

An appetizer can be:

ANTIPASTO: A course of appetizers in an Italian meal

CANAPÉ: An appetizer consisting usually of a thin slice of bread or toast spread with caviar or cheese or other savory food.

COCKTAIL: An alcoholic drink consisting of a spirit or spirits mixed with other ingredients such as a fruit juice or cream, or a dish consisting of small pieces of food, typically served as an hors d'oeuvres e.g., a "prawn cocktail" served as a first course of a meal.

HORS D'OEUVRES (STARTER): A dish served as an appetizer before the main meal.

CRUDITÉS: Raw vegetables cut into bite-sized strips and served with a dip.

APERITIF: An alcoholic drink taken before a meal to stimulate the appetite.

SOUPS AND CONSOMMÉS

VEGETABLE SALAD

SECOND COURSE MEAL

MAIN COURSE This is the most important course and usually the largest. Entrée refers to the main course of a meal, which is a heavy meat course in North American English (USA and parts of Canada). In France the entrée is the course that precedes the main course in a three-course meal or between two principal courses of a meal.

THIRD COURSE MEAL

DESSERT: It is the sweet course eaten at the end of a meal. A dessert can take the form of tarts, cakes, pies, fresh fruits, puddings, ice creams, biscuits, custards, cookies, gelatins, pastries, sweet soups, soufflés, sorbets, sherbets, and dessert wines such as sherry.

SIX-WEEK DAILY MENU PLANNING

FIRST WEEK

DAYS	BREAKFAST	LUNCH	DINNER
MONDAY	Beverage Corn Pap / Beans Akra Paw paw	Corn Foo foo Smoked Fish Njama-Njama Soup Meat Stew Fruit Salad.	Plain Boiled Rice Beef Tomato Stew Sauté Courgette Orange
TUESDAY	Beverage Dodo / Omelet Orange Juice	Boiled White Yams / Ndole Soup Watermelon Meat Balls	Spaghetti Meat Balls in Gravy Paw Paw
WEDNESDAY	Beverage Quaker Oats Soft Boiled Eggs Carrot Juice	Boiled Cocoyams / Bean Soup Mixed Vegetable Salad Banana	Boiled Ripe Plantains Fresh Fish Pepper Soup Cucumber in Vinegar Mango
THURSDAY	Beverage Toast / Scrambled Eggs Grapefruit	Perfumed Rice/Catfish Mbongo Chobi Mixed Salad Pineapple	Yellow Yams Basque Chicken Tomato/Onions/Green Pepper Salad Orange
FRIDAY	Beverage Fried Irish Potatoes Fried Eggs Lemon Drink	Water Foofoo / Eru Soup Carrot Salad Tangerine	Boiled Plantains African Eggplant Stew Fruit Salad Cake
SATURDAY	Beverage Puff Puff / Beans Stew Orange	Equacoco Ya Mosaka/Mbanga Soup Cabbage Salad Mango	Boiled Sweet Potatoes Delicious Groundnut Stew Marinated Tomatoes Pawpaw
SUNDAY	Beverage Corn Flakes Boiled Eggs Watermelon	Basmati Rice/Dijon Chicken Madras Salad Banana	Dodo /Egusi Cabbage Soup Cucumber Mint Salad Pineapple

SECOND WEEK

DAYS	BREAKFAST	LUNCH	DINNER
MONDAY	Beverage Quaker Oats Soft Boiled Eggs Orange	Boiled White Yams/Amaranth Soup Herbs Beetroot Salad Watermelon	Garri FooFoo / Beef Okro Soup Paw Paw
TUESDAY	Beverage Corn Flakes Roast African Plum Grapefruit Juice	Esuba /Egusi Bitter Leaf Soup Cole Slaw Mango	Boiled Cassava Foot Cow Pepper Soup Cabbage Salad Pineapple
WEDNESDAY	Beverage Corn Pap/Banana Akra Lemon Drink	Corn Foo Foo /Kahtti Katthi Sauce Crispy Njama-Njama Fruit Salad	Miondo Rolls/Grilled Fish Sauté Sweet Pepper Watermelon
THURSDAY	Beverage French Bread Scrambled Eggs Paw Paw	White Rice/ Dijon Chicken Sauté Carrots Orange	Dodo/Beef Curry Red Cabbage Salad Grapefruit
FRIDAY	Beverage PuffPuff/Sauté Mushrooms Tangerine	Pounded Plantains/ Chicken Egusi Soup Cucumber Salad Pineapple	Corn Pudding / Vegetable Curry Fresh Fish Stew Mango
SATURDAY	Beverage Akra Beans/Millet Pap Oranges	Rice Foo Foo / Egusi Okro Soup Country Njama Njama Fruit Salad.	Corn Koki Super Salad Bread Paw Paw
SUNDAY	Beverage Fried Irish Potatoes / Omelet Tomato Juice	Perfumed Rice / Chicken CEO Tessas Sauté Veggies Apple	Boiled Irish Potatoes/ Beer Beef Stew Mint Cucumber Grapefruit

THIRD WEEK

DAYS	BREAKFAST	LUNCH	DINNER
MONDAY	Beverage French Toast Roast Plums Orange	Plain Boiled White Rice Mummy's Curry Chicken Tessa's Sauté Veggies Pineapple	Boiled Yellow Yams Palm Oil Pili-Pili Capitaine Vegetable Salad Paw Paw
TUESDAY	Beverage Pancakes Boiled Eggs Grapefruit Juice	Boiled Spaghetti /Ratatouille Watermelon	Boiled Irish Potatoes Onion Livers Beetroot/Onion Salad Mango
WEDNESDAY	Beverage Dodo / Scrambled Eggs Lemon Drink	Achu Foo Foo/Yellow Soup Crispy Njama-Njama Fruit Salad.	Boiled Rice/ Chicken DG Yoghurt Cabbage Salad Grapefruit.
THURSDAY	Beverage Quaker Oats Hard Boiled Eggs Orange Juice	Sese Plantains Tomato/French Bean Salad Mango	Boiled Potatoes Fish Pepper Soup Cucumber Salad
FRIDAY	Beverage Corn Pap /Akra Beans Tangerine.	Corn Chaff Marinated Tomatoes Orange	Boiled Plantains African Eggplant Stew Paw Paw
SATURDAY	Beverage Fried Irish Potatoes Stewed Beef Liver PawPaw	Equacoco À Vekoo Sauté Green Peppers Watermelon	Bobolo/Miondo /Mpub Fish Sauté Cucumber Banana
SUNDAY	Beverage Puff-Puff / Bean Stew Carrot Juice	Boiled Cocoyams /Chicken Egusi Soup Vegetable Salad Pineapple	Dodo / Chicken Dijon Sauté Amaranth Fruit Salad.

FOURTH WEEK

DAYS	BREAKFAST	LUNCH	DINNER
MONDAY	Beverage Quaker Oats Hard Boiled Eggs Orange	Corn Foo Foo / Nkwi Soup Folong Au Poisson Fume Watermelon	Boiled Noodles / Braised Steak Mixed Vegetables Pineapple
TUESDAY	Beverage Fried Irish Potatoes Omelet Lemon Drink	Dodo/Bean Stew Crispy Njama-Njama Lettuce Salad Banana	Boiled Cassava / Njangsa Fish Stew Marinated Tomatoes Mango
WEDNESDAY	Beverage Dodo / Dijon Kidney Tangerine	Perfumed Rice / Chicken Fricassee Sauté Cucumber Orange	Boiled Sweet Potatoes Groundnut Soup/Spiced Cauliflower Grapefruit
THURSDAY	Beverage Fettucine Meat Balls Curry Carrot Juice	Boiled Ripe Plantains / Beef/Potato Stew Beet Root Salad Pawpaw	Boiled White Yam Mona Style Beef Cabbage Mint Cucumber Pineapple
FRIDAY	Beverage Corn Pap /Banana Akra Orange Juice	Boiled Cassava / Beans Koki Mint Salad Apple	Ununu/Fresh Fish Pepper Soup Red Cabbage Curry Mango
SATURDAY	Beverage Toast Sausage Sauté Green Pepper Pineapple	Boiled Yellow Yams / Jamaican Casserole Cole Slaw Banana	Boiled Noodles / Goulash Vinegar Braised Beet Root Grapefruits
SUNDAY	Beverage French Bread /Sardine Omelet Grapefruit.	Jollof Rice Mixed Vegetable Salad Watermelon	Spaghetti Bordelaise Mushroom Tomato/Onions/Green Beans Salad Paw Paw

FIFTH WEEK

DAYS	BREAKFAST	LUNCH	DINNER
MONDAY	Beverage Fried Irish Potatoes / Omelet Apple	Achu Foo Foo /Chi Na'a/ Ndzap Pineapple Fried Fish	Miondo Rolls / Poisson Braise Sauté Carrots Orange
TUESDAY	Beverage Bean Stew/Puff Puff Tangerine	Millet Foo Foo Lalo Soup/zom non amér Mint Cucumber Banana	Boiled Plantains Bewole sauté aux crevettes. Red Cabbage Salad Watermelon
WEDNESDAY	Beverage Millet Pap / Beans Akra Paw Paw	Boiled White Yams / Kpwem Sans Sel Mixed Vegetable Salad Mango	Boiled Rice / Zalam Zalaina Tomato/Onion/Green Pepper Salad Apple
THURSDAY	Beverage Quaker Oats Soft Boiled Eggs Lemon Drink	Bobolo/Okok Sauté Green Peppers Fruit Salad	Macabo Ma Sese Yogurt Cabbage Salad Pineapple
FRIDAY	Beverage Dodo/Liver Stew Grapefruit	Boiled Cassava / Fish Ndomba Sauté Veggies Orange	Miondo/Bobolo / Nnam Owondo Simple Vegetable Salad Watermelon
SATURDAY	Beverage Corn Flakes Poached Eggs Orange Juice	Beef Kondre Cabbage Salad Banana	Ekwang Pottage Madras Salad Pawpaw
SUNDAY	Beverage French Bread / Sausage Passion Fruit Juice	Boiled Yams / Nfian Ngon Herbs/Beetroot Salad Pineapple	Boiled Plantains Patte de boeuf Pepe Soup (Foot cow Pepper Soup) Cucumber Salad Orange.

SIXTH WEEK

DAYS	BREAKFAST	LUNCH	DINNER
MONDAY	**Beverage Quaker Oats Boiled Eggs Grapefruit**	**Rice Foo Foo /Wosangu Mpiank-Nouak Soup Paw Paw**	**Boiled Cassava Efirge Zong/zom non amér Fruit Salad**
TUESDAY	**Beverage Dodo/Dijon Kidney Orange Juice**	**Ntouba Ekon / Mendim Me Zong Beef Soya Pineapple**	**Pounded Cocoyams Assok Bitatam Vegetable Salad Mango**
WEDNESDAY	**Beverage Toast/ Sardine Omelet Paw Paw**	**Nkum-Nkum Okporoko/Agbono Soup Cucumber Salad Banana**	**Bobolo/Miondo Le Sanga'a / Sauté Veggies Watermelon**
THURSDAY	**Beverage Scotch Eggs Corn Flakes Lemon Drink**	**Banane Malaxee Super Salad Watermelon**	**Boiled Yellow Yams/Ossang Fish Stew Paw Paw**
FRIDAY	**Beverage Puff Puff /Sauté Liver Pineapple Juice**	**Ekoka Makwamba Mixed Vegetable Salad Mango**	**Boiled Plantains Folon aux poissons fumés Grapefruit**
SATURDAY	**Beverage Fried Irish Potatoes/ Bean Stew Orange**	**Ndengue /Meukeleu Boulettes De Viande Au Boeuf Et Porc Banana**	**Millet Foo Foo / Sauté Fii Gbarak A Tien Fruit Salad**
SUNDAY	**Beverage Vermicelles Meat Balls in Gravy Grapefruit Juice**	**Boiled Cocoyams / Poisson Sauce Njangsa Sauté Carrots Watermelon**	**Macabo Rape Sauce Gumbo à la viande Mixed Vegetable Salad Paw Paw**

RECEPTION MENUS

For reception menus choose from each table as follows: 2 Carbohydrate dishes, 2 vegetables dishes, 1 meat dish, 1 fish dish, 1 poultry dish, 1 salad dish 1 dessert (fresh fruit, cake, fruit salad, or any sweet dish.) You may have about a total of 9 dishes for a reception.

MENUS FOR LUNCHEONS OR DINNER BANQUET PARTIES		
Boiled Irish potatoes Fried Rice Pottage Crispy njama – njama Sauté Courgette Basque chicken Sauté Tripe Crevettes á la Sawa Mixed Salad Pawpaw	Perfumed Rice Ekwang pottage Mona style Beef cabbage Sauté Cucumber Fried Fish Egg Ratatouille Beetroot/Onion Salad Watermelon	Jollof rice Boiled White Yams Ndole Soup Sauté pork Fried Chicken Fried Fish Super Salad Tessa Sauté Veggies Plain cake
Boiled Yellow Yams Boiled Green Plantains Dijon Kidneys Curry Chicken Bewolé Sauté á la Sawa Mpub fish Cold slaw Pineapple	Bobolo/ Miondo Coconut Rice Egusi Pudding Sauté Liver Ossang Soup Grilled Fish Chicken Fricassee Red Cabbage Salad Oranges	White Boiled Rice Equacoco á Vekoo Tomato Stew Vegetable Curry Sauté Beef Trotters Fish Ndomba Roast Chicken Cucumber Salad Fruit Salad
Achu Foo foo Bekwan / Bekwong **Yellow soup** **Folong au Poisson fumé** **Fried fish** **Fried chicken**	**Water foofoo** **Boiled ripe plantain Eru/okok/ Ikok** **Dijon kidneys** **Fish stew** **Glazed carrots**	**Jollof rice** **Dodo** **Fried njama – njama** **Mummy's porcupine** **Roast fish** **Fried chicken**
Carrot Salad **Madras sald** **Watermelon**	**Sauté Goat** **Mint cucumber Pawpaw**	**Glazed carrots** **Mixed Green salad** **Pineapple**

RECIPE

A recipe is a set of instructions that describes how to prepare or make something, especially a culinary dish. It is a set of instructions for preparing a particular dish including a list of the ingredients required

COMPONENTS OF A RECIPE

1. The name (and often the local name or origin) of the dish.
2. How much time it will take to prepare the dish.
3. The required ingredients along with their quantities or proportions.
4. Necessary equipment and environment needed to prepare the dish.
5. An ordered list of preparation steps and techniques
6. The number of servings that the recipe will provide (the "yield")
7. The texture and flavor
8. A photograph of the finished dish
9. How long the dish will keep and suitability for freezing
10. Nutritional information, such as calories per serving and grams of protein, fat and carbohydrate per serving may be given.
11. Variations of a traditional dish, if it gives different tastes of the same recipes

BASIC COOKING INGREDIENTS

TYPES OF SALT

Salt is a crystalline mineral made of two elements sodium (Na) and Chlorine.

KOSHER SALT: It is called kosher because it is useful for the Jewish people. Kosher salt has a flaky, coarse structure. Used for all cooking and it dissolves fast, and its flavor disperses quickly. It is none iodized.

REGULAR TABLE SALT (REFINED SALT): This is the most commonly used salt. This salt is highly refined and heavily ground, with most of the impurities and trace minerals are removed. Anti-caking agents are added so that it flows freely. Iodine is often added to table salt and it is almost pure sodium chloride, at 97% or higher.

SEA SALT: It is made by evaporating sea water. It is mostly just sodium chloride. It is similar to regular salt but can contain small amounts of minerals.

ROCK SALT: Large, chunky, non-uniform crystals. Used for making ice cream and deicing.

PICKLING SALT: Very fine grained, like table salt. Used for brining pickles and sauerkraut and non-iodized.

FLEUR DE SEL: Used for a special-occasion table salt. It is crystalline which melts slowly in the mouth. It is a hand harvested sea salt.

LOSALT: A salt substitute containing potassium chloride in addition to sodium chloride. In Cameroon there is **FAITOUT** which is a salt substitute.

TYPES OF MILK & MILK PRODUCTS

WHOLE MILK: It has the highest percentage of fat in it, around 3.8% on average. Full cream milk has the creamiest taste due to the higher fat content.

LOW FAT: It has slightly less fat in it, around 1.3% to 1.4%

SKIMMED MILK: It has the lowest amount of fat in it with no more than 0.15% milk fat.

LACTOSE-FREE MILK: This is regular milk that has been processed to break down lactose (sugar) in it so as to help people with lactose intolerance to easily digest milk.

SOY MILK: made from soya beans.

BUTTERMILK: Buttermilk is fresh milk with an added bacterial culture (similar to yogurt) that gives it a tangy flavor and thick, rich texture. It adds tenderness to baked goods, and a light, tangy flavor to soups and salads.

EVAPORATED MILK: About 60% of water is evaporated from fresh skim milk, 2% from whole milk. Evaporated milk is sealed in cans and is heat tolerant, making it suitable for baked goods and slow-cooker recipe e.g., Liquid peak milk

SWEETENED CONDENSED MILK: Milk made commercially by condensing milk to 1/3 of its original volume and then sugar is added. It is a sweetened condensed milk, very thick and sweet and is available in cans. It is most often used in sweet baked goods and it is not interchangeable with other types of milk.

POWDERED MILK (SKIM OR WHOLE MILK POWDER) DRIED: Partly evaporated milk is heated and dried instantly e.g., powdered peak milk etc. Powdered milk is made from whole or skim milk and is available in bags and in bulk. There are instant and regular formulas. Once the package is opened it should be used within a month.

UHT (ULTRA HIGH TEMPERATURE) MILK: Sterilized milk that has been heat-treated at an ultra-high temperature (138 to 150$^{oC).}$ Once it has cooled down, the milk is poured into a sterilized package without air contact, usually a Tetra pak type box. Unopened UHT milk keeps for several months at room temperature. Once opened, it must be refrigerated and consumed within 3 days.

RAW OR UNPASTEURIZED MILK: This is milk that has not been pasteurized. It may contain bacteria that can cause serious illnesses, such as tuberculosis. Pasteurization destroys 100% of pathogenic bacteria, yeast and mold and 95% to 99% of other bacteria.

PARTLY SKIMMED MILKS/SEMI SKIMMED: It is the most popular types of milk for everyday use. When a portion of milk fat is removed it becomes partly skimmed milk, such as 2% milk and 1% milk depending on the quantity removed. Skim milk is fat-free, with only 0.1% fat. They contain 16 essential nutrients.

YOGURT

DEFINITION: Yogurt is a prepared food having the consistency of custard, made from milk curdled by the action of cultures, sometimes sweetened or flavored. It is a solid sour like food prepared from milk fermented by added bacteria known as yogurt cultures. Milk used for yogurt can be homogenized or not.

VARIETIES OF YOGURT

1. Sweetened and flavored yogurt
2. Strained yogurt
3. Beverages: Drinking or drinkable yogurt, Yogurt smoothies, Yogurt soup (yogurt + rice + flour + dried mint), Plant-milk yogurt (soy milk, rice milk and nut milk such as almond milk and coconut. The most widely sold variety of plant milk yogurt is soy yogurt. These yogurts are suitable for vegans, and people with intolerance to dairy milk and those who prefer plant milks.

CREAM

Cream is the thick white or pale-yellow fatty liquid which rises to the top when milk is left to stand, and which can be eaten as an accompaniment to desserts or used as a cooking ingredient. It is also called **sweet cream**.

Cream has a higher butter fat layer skimmed from the top of milk before homogenization. Cream can be dried and exported.

Cream is classified by its butterfat content as follows:

1. **LIGHT CREAM ALSO CALLED TABLE CREAM:** 18-30% fat used for soups, **sauces** and garnishes for desserts such as fresh fruit.
2. **LIGHT WHIPPING CREAM:** 30-36% fat, used for sauces, soups, garnishing of desserts, and used for whipped cream.
3. **HEAVY CREAM:** 36% fat, used for whipped cream for better peaks. It is used for making Crème fraîche and sour cream, which contains 10-45% butterfat with bacterial culture. In French, it is also called crème **fraîche epaisse**, **fermentée, crème fraîche liquid,** or **Fleurette**. Crème fraiche is used as basis of desserts and dessert sauces. Cream is used in many foods such as ice cream, many sauces soups, stews, puddings, and some custard bases and cakes. Whipped cream is served as a topping on ice cream, sundaes, milk shakes, egging, and sweet pies. The word crème denotes not only dairy cream but also other thick liquids such as sweet and savory custards, which are normally made with milk, not cream.

CHEESE

Cheese is a food derived from milk that is produced in a wide range of flavors, textures, and forms by coagulation of the milk protein casein. It comprises protein and fat from milk, usually milk of cows, buffalo, goats, or sheep.

TYPES OF CHEESE: There are many types of cheese, from 400, 500, or 1000 by different federations or groups.

Varieties may be grouped or classified according to these criteria: Length of aging, texture, methods of making, fat content, animal milk, country, or region of origin, etc.

These criteria are used singly or in combination, but with no single method being used universally. The method most traditionally used is based on **moist content**, which is then further discriminated by **fat content,** by curing or ripening methods:

MOISTURE CONTENT: Soft, semi-soft, semi-hard, hard, fresh, whey and stretched cured cheeses. Age of the cheese; Fresh cheese without preservatives can spoil within a number of days.

FAT CONTENT: (double cream, goat, ewe, and water buffalo)

Most of the world's commercially available cheese is made from cow's milk. Double cream cheeses are soft cheeses, of cow's milk enriched with cream so that their fat content is 60%. A triple cream is 75%. The content of whole cow's milk is 3%- 4%, so the double cream or triple cream is not a quantitative reference to the change in fat content.

SOFT-RIPENED AND BLUE-VEIN: The presence of mold soft ripened cheeses, washed rind cheeses, and blue cheeses.

PROCEEDED CHEESES: It is made from traditional cheeses and emulsifying salts, often with the addition of milk, more salt preservatives, and food coloring. It is inexpensive, consistent, and melts smoothly. It is sold packaged and either pre-sliced or unsliced, in a number of varieties.

It is also available in some countries in aerosol cans. Some popular cow cheeses are camembert, cotija, mozzarella, Emmental, cheddar, Gouda, Taleggio, Parmigiano – Reggiano and Monterey Jack. Chevre is goat cheese known is France as fromage de chevre. Roquefort, Feta and Manchego are sheep cheese

BUTTER

Whole butter is a mixture of fats, milk solids, and moisture derived by churning cream until the oil droplets stick together and can be separated out. Used for baking and cooking.

BUTTER (GHEE) CLARIFIED: Has a higher smoking point than butter. Used for frying and sautéing.

ICE CREAM

Ice cream is a soft, sweet, frozen, food made from cream or milk and butter fat, sugar, flavorings such as vanilla or chocolate, and sometimes eggs and fruits. It is a dessert and a snack and can be served in dishes for eating with a spoon, or in cones, which are licked. Ice cream may be served with other desserts, such as apple pie and also used to prepare other desserts such as ice cream floats, milk shakes, sundaes, and baked Alaska.

ICE CREAM-LIKE FROZEN DESSERTS

1. **FROZEN CUSTARD**: At least 10% milk fat and at least 1.4% egg yolk.
2. **FROZEN YOGURT:** Made with yogurt instead of milk or cream.
3. **GELATO:** An Italian frozen dessert with a lower fat content than ice cream.
4. **POPSICLE:** (Ice pop or ice lolly): Frozen fruit purée, fruit juice, or flavored sugar on a stick or in a flexible plastic sleeve.
5. **SHERBET:** 1-2% milk fat and sweeter than ice cream.
6. **SORBET:** Fruit puree with no dairy products.
7. **Flavored sugar water on a stick or in a plastic** bag is usually called **ALASKA** in Cameroon.

VARIETIES OF SUGAR/SUGAR SUBSTITUTES

GRANULATED SUGAR: It is highly refined, multipurpose, made from sugarcane and sugar beets. It is also called refined, table or white sugar. It is the commonest type of sugar used in baking and cooking. Has coarser crystals.

CASTER SUGAR (CASTOR SUGAR): Superfine granulated white sugar. The crystals are so fine, thus dissolve much quicker than standard granulated white sugar. It is ideal for making meringues, syrups, and cocktails because it dissolves quickly, icings, confections and whipping cream.

CONFECTIONERS SUGAR: It is a type of white sugar that has been ground into a fine powder. A small amount (3%) of cornstarch is blended in so as to avoid caking or clumping. It easily dissolves in liquid. It is ideal for making icing and frosting, as well as decorating baked goods.

It is also referred to as powdered sugar and 10 x sugar. In Canada and Great Britain, it is called Icing sugar and in France Sucre glace.

PEARL SUGAR/COARSE SUGAR OR DECORATING SUGAR: It is a variety of white sugar that has a course, hard texture, and an opaque color. It also holds its shape and doesn't melt when exposed to high temperatures. It is also called Nib sugar or hail sugar and commonly used in Scandinavian baking to decorate pastries, cookies, and buns. Used in making fondants, confections, and liquors.

SANDING SUGAR (COARSE SUGAR): It has large crystals which are resistant to heat. Sanding sugar is used mainly for decorating which adds extra texture and crunch to cookies and other baked goods. It is available in many colors. It is used as a sprinkle on top of baked goods. The large crystals reflect light and give the product a sparkling appearance.

CANE SUGAR: It is produced solely from sugar cane. It has a slightly large grain, darker color and it is more expensive. It is used the same way as for granulated sugar.

DEMERARA SUGAR (BOJET BROWN SUGAR): It is a variety of raw cane sugar that is minimally refined. It has large grains with an amber color and a natural, subtle molasses flavor. Demerara sugar is used to sweeten coffee or tea, or as a topping on baked goods like muffins, scones, cookies, and cakes. It is popular in England. It is a light brown sugar with golden crystals, which are slightly sticky from the adhering molasses.

TURBINADOR: A minimally refined raw cane sugar, has large medium brown crystals, and is often mistaken for standard brown sugar because of its color. It has a delicate caramel flavor and is often used to sweeten beverage and can also be used in baking.

MUSCOVADO SUGAR: It is a variety of unrefined cane sugar in which the molasses is not removed. It comes in dark and light varieties, and has a sticky, wet, sandy texture with a rich, complex flavor. It can be used as a substitute for brown sugar. It is used in barbecue sauce, marinades, and savory dishes. It is referred to as Barbados sugar. It is a British specialty.

LIGHT BROWN SUGAR: This is refined white sugar with a small amount of molasses added in. It has a wet, sandy texture, less sticky than muscovado sugar and a delicate caramel flavor. It is used for making any baked goods, as well as in savory goods, butterscotch condiments, and glazes.

DARK BROWN SUGAR: It is also refined white sugar with molasses added. It contains more molasses than light brown sugar which gives it a stronger, more intense flavor. Light and dark brown sugar can be used interchangeably. It can be used in gingerbread, minced meat, baked beans, and other full-flavored goods.

ARTIFICIAL SWEETENERS AND SUGAR SUBSTITUTES

SUCROSE found naturally in fruit added to baked goods, jams, marinades, salad dressings.

ACESULFAME POTASSIUM:

Found in soft drinks, gelatins, chewing gum, frozen desserts.

AGAVE NECTAR: Found in cereals, yogurts, tea

ASPARTAME: Found in drinks, gum, yogurt, cough drops

HIGH-FRUCTOSE CORN SYRUP: Found in sodas, desserts cereals.

HONEY: Found in cereals, baked goods, and teas.

NEOTAME: Found in some drinks, dairy products, frozen desserts, puddings, and fruit juices.

STEVIA LEAF EXTRACT: Found in drinks, yogurts, individual packets.

SACCHARIN: Found in drinks, canned goods, candy

SUCRALOSE: Found in fruit drinks canned fruit, and syrup

SUGAR ALCOHOLS: Found in sugar free candies, gum, desserts.

TYPES OF COOKING OIL

LIGHT, PURE OR REGULAR OLIVE OIL: It is light in color and taste not calories than straight Evoo. It has a smoking point of 465-470oF which makes it ideal for high-heat cooking. It can be used in vinaigrettes. Light Olive oil is treated with chemicals to neutralize the color.

EXTRA VIRGIN OLIVE OIL (EVOO): It's robust in flavor, and can have buttery, spicy, fruity, or grassy notes depending on the Olives point of origin. Evoo's lower smoke point (about 325°) means it is not great for cooking. It is good for vinaigrettes, ice cream and finishing oil.

PEANUT OIL: It is pale yellow in color, with a nutty scent and powerful flavor. It can go rancid quickly, so store in a cool dry place, and use it within a few months. The smoke point is 450oF, so it is recommended for high-heat cooking, frying, and salad dressings.

PALM OIL: It is a saturated fat made from the palm tree. It is semi-solid at room temperature and very efficient in frying with a smoke point of just below 450oF. A yellowish - orange fatty oil used for cooking flavoring.

CORN OIL: Its smoking points is 450oF, thus good for frying especially refined corn oil. It has a neutral flavor and is used frequently in commercial kitchens. A mild medium yellow color refined oil. It is made from the germ of the corn kernel and used for frying, salad dressings, and shortening.

COCONUT OIL: It is solid at room temperature, which means it's not ideal for vinaigrettes or as finishing oil. It is good for moderate-heat roasting. Its smoking point is 350oF. It melts and gives off a tropical scent when heated. It is similar to butter consistency when cold makes it good for non-dairy baked goods. It is heavy, nearly colorless. Used for coatings, confectionary, shortening.

VEGETABLE OIL: It is typically a blend of many different refined oils is neutral tasting and smelling and has a smoke point of about 400oF. It is good for high heat sauteing and frying, salad dressing.

CANOLA OIL: It is pressed from the rapeseed plant, and it is similar to vegetable oil in flavor, color, and smoke point and usage qualities. Canola oil and vegetable oil can be used in salad dressings. It will go rancid in about a year. It should be stored in a cool, dark place, away from the stovetop and oven. It is light, golden-colored oil. Good all-purpose oil used in cooking.

GRAPE SEED OIL: It is light green in color with a smoke point of 420oF. It is clean, plays-well-with-others taste and often used in vinaigrettes because it is less expensive than **Evoo. It is a by-product of wine making. Good for sautéing or frying, and salad dressings.**

AVOCADO OIL: It is high in monounsaturated fat, has a smoke point of about 520oF, which makes it an efficient pantry item. It is used for sautéing, roasting, searing and vinaigrettes. It should be stored in a cool, dark cupboard. It is vibrant green in color with a soft, nutty taste and mild avocado aroma.

SUNFLOWER OIL:

It is light, odorless, and nearly flavorless oil. It has a smoke point of 440-450oF is the pantry hero for all things sear-and sauté-related. It does turn rancid quicker than other oils because it is pressed from seeds, so store in a cool place and use within a year maximum Used for cooking, margarine, salad dressings and shortening.

SESAME OIL: It has a smoke point of 410oF and a neutral flavor. It is great general-purpose oil used for sautés, roasts, and others. It should be stored in a cool cupboard.

HEMP SEED OIL: It has a very nutty, rich flavor and dark green color. It is too sensitive to be heated. Use as finishing oil for soups or grain bowls. Store it in the refrigerator.

Flaxseed oil: It is also nutty tasting, but too much can impart a fishy, funky flavor. Use sparingly in dressings or as a finisher. Keep in the fridge.

TOASTED NUT AND SEED OILS (WALNUT, PISTACHIOS SESAME, ETC): They are delicate in smoke point. (Don't heat them at oil) but they're big on flavor.

SOYBEAN OIL: It is a vegetable oil extracted from the seeds of the soybean (Glycine max). It is one of the most widely consumed cooking oils. Soybean oil is used in salad dressing, mayonnaise, bread, margarine, sandwich, spreads, non-dairy coffee creamers, snack foods. The high smoke point of soybean 450oF makes it good for frying. Store in a dry and dark place and shelf life is one year at room temperature. Soybean oil is a fairly heavy oil with a pronounced flavor and aroma.

SAFFLOWER: A golden color with light texture oil. Used for margarine, mayonnaise, salad dressing.

ALMOND OIL: It has a subtle toasted almond aroma and flavor used in sauce and stir fry for Asian food.

COTTON SEED OIL: Pale-yellow oil that is extracted from the seed of the cotton plant. Used for margarine, salad dressings, shortening and for frying.

HAZELNUT OIL: Used in salad dressings, marinades, and baked goods.

MACADAMIA OIL (NUT OIL): Cold pressed from the decadent macadamia nut similar in quality to the finest extra virgin olive oil. Used for sauté, pan fry, sear, deep fry, stir fry, grill, broil, and baking.

RICH BRAN OIL: Used for frying, sauté, salad dressings, baking and dipping oil

WALNUT OIL: medium-yellow oil with a nutty flavor and aroma. More perishable than most other oils. Used for sauté, panfry, sear, deep fry, stir fry, grill, boil.

COOKING FAT

BUTTER: Whole butter is a mixture of fats, milk solids, and moisture derived by churning cream until the oil droplets stick together and can be separated out. Used for baking and cooking.

BUTTER (GHEE) CLARIFIED: Has a higher smoking point than butter. Used for frying and sautéing.

LARD: This is white solid or semi-solid fat of a hog or pig. Used for baking and frying

SHORTENING: (Vegetable) Blended oil solidified using various processes. Used for baking and frying.

MARGARINE: Provides color and flavor to food.

RAISING AGENTS

BAKING POWDER

KINDS OF BAKING POWDER: Baking powder is bicarbonate of soda + acidic ingredient + cornstarch sometimes and cream of tartar. (2 parts cream of tartar plus 1 part bicarbonate of soda).

DOUBLE-ACTING: It releases leavening gases on contact with moisture and again during baking. This is the most commonly used baking powder.

TARTRATE (CREAM OF TARTAR): A single-acting powder that releases a volume of gas the instant it touches moisture.

PHOSPHATE: A slightly slower-to-act single acting powder.

BAKING SODA

Baking soda is the same as bicarbonate of soda. In the USA it is called Baking soda. In Europe and Africa, it is called Bicarbonate of soda

YEAST

TYPES OF YEAST FOR BAKING

FRESH YEAST: Also known as cake yeast, compressed yeast, in Italian, LIEVITO DI BIRRA FRESCA (fresh beer yeast). It is squidgy and crumbly. In using fresh yeast, you activate in liquid-water or milk if you are doing enriched dough.

Store in the fridge and it will only last for a few weeks maximum.

ACTIVE DRY YEAST (ADY): Have small granules and doesn't need to be stored in the fridge. To activate ADY add it in liquid, add sugar or honey to the liquid. This is the most well-known yeast. It is dissolved in warm water of (about 100F).

INSTANT YEAST: Also known as easy blend, easy-bake yeast, fast action or quick, dry, or dried yeast. It is similar to ADY, but is finer, almost powdery. They come in sachets of 7g which is about 1 1/2 teaspoons. It is not necessary to activate it or mix it with liquid first, you add it directly to the flour. It is the most popular type of yeast.

TYPES OF FLOUR

ALL-PURPOSE FLOUR: It is the most widely used of all flours. It is made from a combination of hard and soft wheat, hence the term all-purpose. It can be used universally for a wide range of baked products, yeast breads, cakes, cookies, and pastries.

BREAD FLOUR: It is milled primarily for commercial baking use, similar to all-purpose flour, but has higher gluten content.

CAKE FLOUR: It is fine-textured, almost silky flour milled from soft wheat and has low protein content. It is used to make all types of baked goods, like cakes, cookies, crackers, quick breads, and some kinds of pastries.

PASTRY FLOUR: Its properties fall between all-purpose flour and cake flour. It is usually made from soft wheat. It can be used for cookies, cakes, crackers, and similar baked products. It has a slightly higher protein content than cake flour and less starch.

SELF-RISING FLOUR: This is a type of all-purpose flour that has salt and a leavening agent added. 1 cup contains 1 ½ teaspoons of baking powder and ½ teaspoon salt. Self-rising flour can be substituted for all-purpose flour in a recipe by reducing salt and baking powder according to these proportions. It is commonly used in biscuits, and quick breads or even cookies, but it is not recommended for yeast breads.

SEMOLINA: This is the coarsely ground endosperm of durum wheat. Durum wheat is the hardest variety of the six classes of wheat and has the highest protein content of all wheat. It is used for making high quality pasta, couscous in Africa. It is rarely used to make bread.

DURUM FLOUR: It is a by-product in the production of semolina. It is usually enriched with four B vitamins and iron and used to make noodles.

WHOLE WHEAT FLOUR: This is milled from the entire kernel of wheat. The presence of bran reduces gluten development; therefore, items baked with whole wheat flour tend to be heavier and denser than those made from enriched flour. Bakers add gluten to counteract this (one tablespoon per cup of whole wheat flour is used.

OAT FLOUR: It is gluten-free flour, making it popular for dieters who prefer to avoid gluten

CARAMEL

Caramel is a sugar or syrup heated until it turns brown, used as flavoring or coloring for food or drink. It is a liquid made by cooking until it changes color, used for coloring and flavoring food.

CARAMELIZE To heat sugar until it liquefies and become clear caramel syrup, ranging in color from golden to dark brown. Fruits and vegetable with natural sugars can be caramelized by sautéing, roasting or grilling thereby giving them a sweeter, flavor and golden glaze.

SYRUP

Syrup is a thick sweet liquid made by dissolving sugar in boiling water, often used for preserving fruit. It is a thick sticky solution of sugar and water often flavored or medicated. Syrup is also the concentrated juice of a fruit or a plant. Simple syrups are used to sweeten and/or flavor beverages like tea and cocktail. It is used for baking cakes, marinades, salads, and cooked vegetables.

PUREE

It is a smooth cream of liquidized or crushed fruit or vegetable. A purée or mash is cooked food, usually vegetables or legumes that has been ground, pressed, blended, or sieved to the consistency of a soft creamy paste or thick liquid.

Couli is a French term more commonly used for fruit purees. Purées must be cooked, either before or after grinding in order to improve flavor and texture, remove toxic substances, and/or reduce their water content.

Common purées: common purées include apples, plums and other fruits smashed or mashed for their juice content. Apple purée (Apple sauce), Carrots, Potato (Mashed potatoes), Cassava, Pumpkin, Tomato, Sweet corn.

ROUX

Roux is a mixture of butter and flour used to thicken sauces. The mixture is made by melting butter and stirring in flour. This is often diluted with milk or stock (broth) and cooked for at least 15 minutes while stirring constantly.

For dark roux, the mixture is cooked until it turns brown before liquid is added. Because this cooking reduces the thickening quality of the flour, the amount of flour should be increased. Roux is the base of all sauces. There is brown roux, golden roux, and white roux. There are five basic sauces with many derivatives. Béchamel sauce, Espagnole sauce, Velouté sauce, Hollandaise sauce, and tomatoes sauce. These are known as the French mother sauces. Brown and white roux is made with butter. White roux is cooked until it turns beige, brown until pale golden.

SAUCES

A sauce is a liquid substance served with food to add moistness and flavor e.g., tomato sauce. A sauce is also any preparation, usually liquid or semi-liquid eaten as a gravy or as a relish accompanying food. Synonyms for sauce are relish, dressing condiments, ketchup, dip, jus, and coulis.

BROWN SAUCE: It is normally dark brown in color. The most popular brown sauce is HP sauce in the UK. It is available in catering services sachets and dispenser bottles in restaurants.

BUTTER SAUCE: A sauce made of butter, water, or broth, and seasonings, thickened with flour, and used as a basic for the making of other sauces. A sauce made of melted butter, often diluted with water, sometimes thickened with flour or egg yolk, or both and seasoned with lemon juice. Butter sauces are Meunière sauce, Beurre manie, Café de Paris. The blending of fat (butter or oil) and water (wine, vinegar, or egg yolk which is more than 50% water). The best-known emulsified sauces are Hollandaise and Mayonnaise. Vinaigrette is a temporary emulsion.

COLD EMULSIFIED SAUCES: a thick emulsion of raw egg and oil such as:

- **Mayonnaise, Chantilly, or Mousseline** is Mayonnaise mixed with whipped cream.
- **Herb Mayonnaise** is Mayonnaise aux fines herbes that is Mayonnaise flavored with green herbs such as chervil, parsley, and tarragon.
- **Rémoulade sauce**: Mayonnaise flavored with chopped gherkins, capers, anchory essence, herbs, onion and/or mustard.
- **Tartar sauce:** Mayonnaise sauce made with hard-boiled egg yolk flavored with chopped onion, chives, and/or chervil. Tartar sauce is served with fish.

HOT EMULSIFIED SAUCES:

- **Hollandaise Sauce:** (sauce hollandaise) A basic hollandaise sauce is thickened with egg yolks, lemon juice, and melted butter.
- **Béarnaise sauce** (sauce béarnaise.) Egg yolks + reduced vinegar + butter.

SWEET SAUCES:

- **Custard**: A sweet yellow sauce made from milk, eggs, and sugar. Also called Crème **Anglaise**.
- **Syrup**: A sweet thick liquid made from sugar and other sweet substances, used as a sauce.
- **Caramel sauces**, fruit sauces.

WHITE SAUCES:
(Sauce Blanche) a sauce of flour, melted butter and milk or cream. "Fish in white Sauce", Béchamel sauce, also known as white sauce, is made from a white roux and milk. Béchamel sauce is a base for a number of other classic sauces with additional ingredients added including:

- **Crème sauce** (heavy cream).
- **Mustard sauce** (prepared mustard seed).
- **Veloute sauce Yogurt sauce.** White sauce or sauce Blanche may also be applied to a simple sauce consisting only of milk and melted butter, without flour or spices.

HOT SAUCE: A spicy sauce or condiment made with chili peppers. Hot sauces are also known as chili sauce or pepper sauce.

- **Tabasco** sauce in North America
- **Peri peri** sauce is a style of piri-piri chili sauce used by **Nando's** chicken fast food restaurants in South Africa.
- **Nali** sauce is a style of piri piri chili sauce in Malawi.
- **"Madeira sauce**" A savory sauce made with Madeira wine and served with meat.

NB: Emulsions: A fine dispersion of minute droplets of one liquid in another in which it is not soluble or miscible. "Oil beaten to an emulsion with a half tablespoonful of vinegar."

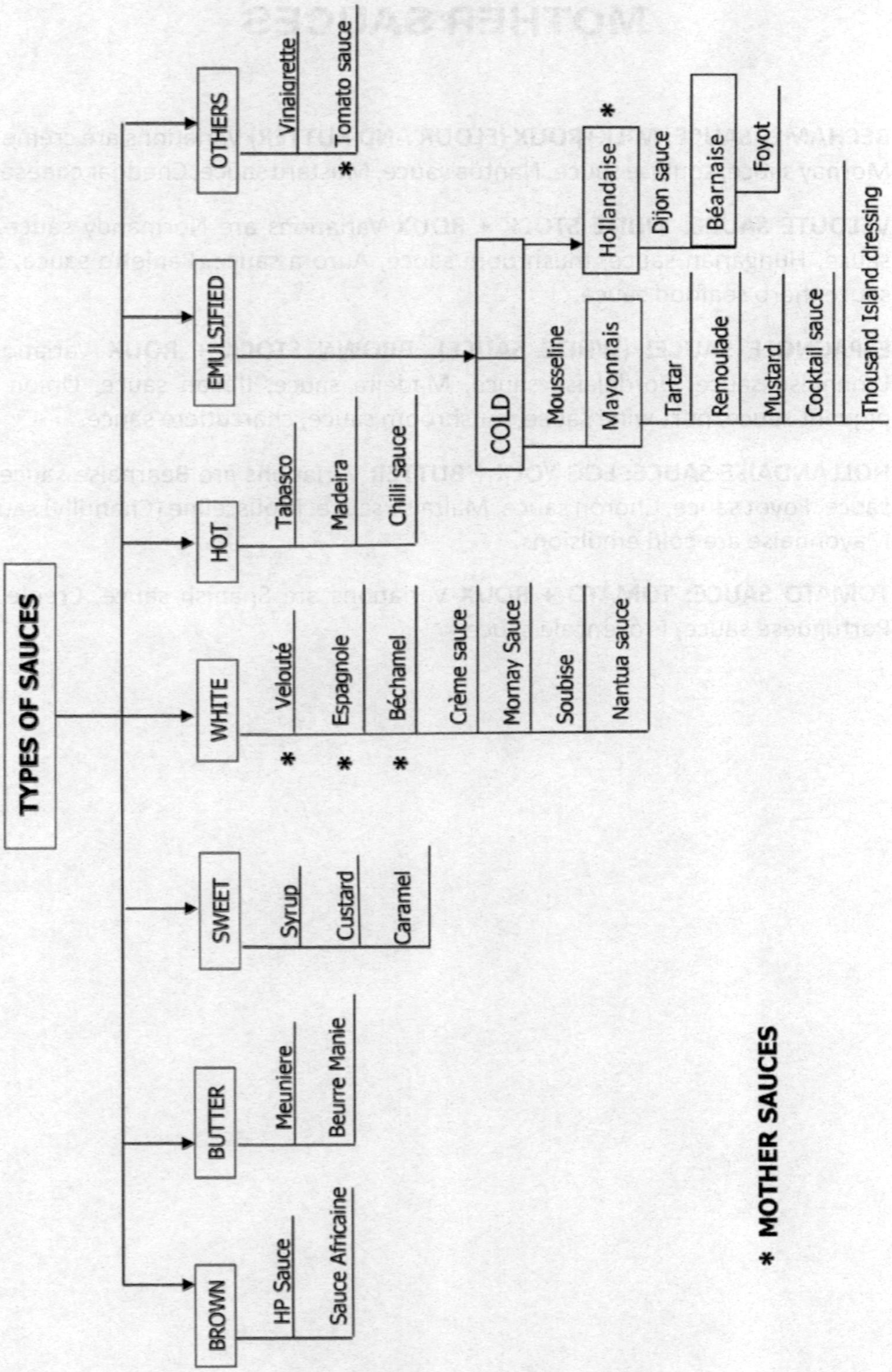
TYPES OF SAUCES
BROWN
HP Sauce
Sauce Africaine
BUTTER
Meuniere
Beurre Manie
SWEET
Syrup
Custard
Caramel
WHITE
* Velouté
* Espagnole
* Béchamel
Crème sauce
Mornay Sauce
Soubise
Nantua sauce
HOT
Tabasco
Madeira
Chilli sauce
EMULSIFIED
COLD
Mousseline
Mayonnais
Tartar
Remoulade
Mustard
Cocktail sauce
Thousand Island dressing
* Hollandaise
Dijon sauce
Béarnaise
Foyot
OTHERS
Vinaigrette
* Tomato sauce
* MOTHER SAUCES

MOTHER SAUCES

1. **BÉCHAMEL SAUCE: MILK+ROUX (FLOUR AND BUTTER)** Variations are crème sauce, Mornay sauce, soubise sauce, Nantua sauce, Mustard sauce, Cheddar cheese sauce.
2. **VELOUTÉ SAUCE: WHITE STOCK + ROUX** Variations are Normandy sauce, Bercy sauce, Hungarian sauce, mushroom sauce, Aurora sauce, Paulette sauce, Shrimp sauce, herb seafood sauce.
3. **ESPAGNOLE SAUCE: (WHITE SAUCE). BROWN STOCK + ROUX** Variations are Lyonnaise sauce, Bordelaise sauce, Madeira sauce, Italian sauce, Onion sauce, piquant sauce, port wine sauce, mushroom sauce, charcutiere sauce.
4. **HOLLANDAISE SAUCE: EGG YOLK + BUTTER** Variations are Bearnaise sauce, Dijon sauce, Foyot sauce, Choron sauce, Maltaise sauce. Mousseline (Chantilly) sauce and Mayonnaise are cold emulsions.
5. **TOMATO SAUCE: TOMATO + ROUX** Variations are Spanish sauce, Creole sauce, Portuguese sauce, Provençale sauce.

FIVE FRENCH MOTHER SAUCES/USES

		Béchamel	Velouté	Espagnole	Hollandaise	Tomato sauce
1	Base	Milk (usually whole milk)	White stock (veal stock, Chicken stock, Fish stock)	Brown sauce (Roasted veal stock, roasted chicken stock.	Egg yolks and Butter.	(Raw tomato paste, tomato purée, stewed tomatoes).
2	Thickening agent	White roux	Roux (sometimes a liaison is used)	Brown roux	Emulsification	Roux
3	Classical flavoring	White onion, clove, bay leaf, salt, white pepper nutmeg.	None	Mirepoix sachet (Bay leaf, Thyme parsley), tomato puree	Pepper corn (black) white wine vinegar, salt, lemon juice, cayenne pepper.	Salt, pork, mirepoix, garlic, white veal stock, pepper, sugar.
4	Common secondary sauces	Cream sauce, Mornay, cheddar cheese sauce, mustard sauce, Nantua	White wine sauce, sauce supreme, sauce Allemande sauce Paulette	Demi-glace, Bordelaise, sauce Robert Lyonnaise, Sauce Madeira, Sauce Bercy, Sauce Chasseur.	Bearnaise, Maltaise Mousseline, Foyot, Choron Mayonnaise	Creole Portuguese and Spanish Sauce tomate
5	Classical served with	Eggs, Fish steamed poultry steamed vegetables, pastas, veal	Eggs, steamed poultry, steamed vegetables pastas, veal.	Meats especially beef, duck, veal, lamb.	Vegetables especially asparagus, eggs, light poultry dishes, fish (Bearnaise sauce)	Pastas, Fish, Vegetables, (especially grilled), potenta veal, poultry (chicken) breads, dumplings.

VINAIGRETTE

Vinaigrette is made by mixing oil with something acidic such as vinegar or lemon juice. The mixture can be enhanced with salt, herbs and/or spices. It is used most commonly as a salad dressing but can also be used as a marinade. Traditionally vinaigrette consists of 3 parts oil and 1 part vinegar mixed into a stable emulsion. Vinaigrette is a diminutive form of the French word vinaigre (vinegar). It was commonly known as "French dressing" in the 19th century.

GELATIN

Gelatin (Gelatine) is a nearly transparent, colorless, or slightly yellowish, brittle, and almost tasteless glutinous substance. It is obtained by boiling ligaments, bones, skin etc. of animals in water. Gelatin forms the basis of jellies, glues etc. The gelatin used to make liquids become firm such as in the making of jelly is a clear and tasteless powder.

USE OF GELATIN

Gelling agent in cooking such as gelatin desserts, marshmallows, and candy corn.

Confections as gummy beers, fruit snacks.

Stabilizer, thickener, texturizer in yogurt, cream cheese, and margarine.

Fat-reduced foods to stimulate the mouth feel of fat and create volume

Production of Chinese soup dumplings

Clarification of juices such as apple juice and vinegar.

JELLY

Jelly is a soft, semi-solid, elastic food substance containing gelatin or pectin etc. from a fruit juice boiled down with sugar and used as a spread for bread and toast, as a filling for cakes or dough nuts etc.

MARSHMALLOW

Marshmallow is a sweet paste or confection made from the mucilaginous root of the marshmallow. It is a soft, sweet, pink, or white food.

SOUFFLÉS

A soufflé is a baked egg-based dish made with egg yolks and beaten egg whites combined with various other ingredients. Soufflé is a French word which means “to breathe” or “to puff”. A soufflé can be a savory main dish or a sweetened dessert

COMPONENTS OF SOUFFLÉS

1. A flavored crème patissière, cream sauce or béchamel or a purée as the base.
2. Egg whites beaten to a soft peak.

The base provides the flavor, and the egg whites provide the “lift” or puffiness to the dish. Herbs, cheese, and vegetables are used to flavor savory souffles. Jam, fruits, berries, chocolate, banana, and lemon are used to flavor dessert soufflés. Soufflés are baked in individual ramekins or other baking vessels. After being cooked, a soufflé is puffed up and fluffy and will generally fall after 5 or 10 minutes.

VARIATIONS OF SOUFFLÉS

1. Savory soufflés include cheese and vegetables such as spinach, carrot, and herbs, and may sometimes incorporate poultry, bacon, ham, or seafood for a more substantial dish.
2. Sweet soufflés may be based on a chocolate or a fruit sauce (lemon or raspberry) for example and often served with a dusting of powdered sugar.
3. Ice cream soufflé, combines a soufflé with ice cream. Fruit or a hot dessert sauce such as chocolate sauce may also be used.

JAM (CONFITURE)

It is a mixture of fruit and sugar that has been cooked and the water evaporates leaving a concentrated mixture of fruit and sugar. A method of preserving fruits.

MARMALADE

A clear jellylike preserve made from the pulp and rind of fruit especially citrus fruits. The pulp of fruit with sugar + ½ the weight of the fruit.

SOUP

Soup is a liquid, typically savory and made by boiling meat, fish, or vegetables etc. in stock or water. It is liquid food generally served warm (but may be cool or cold).

Soups are similar to stews, and in some cases, there may not be a clear distinction between the two; however, soups generally have more liquid than stews. Soups are classified into two groups clear soups and thick soups. Bouillon and consommé are the French classification of soups. Thick soups are classified depending upon the type of thickening agent used:

1. **PURÉE**: vegetables soups thickened with starch
2. **BISQUES**: puréed shellfish or vegetables that is thickened with cream.
3. **CREAM SOUPS**: Thickened with béchamel sauce.
4. **VELOUTES**: Thickened with eggs, butter, and cream. Rice, lentils, flour and grains, carrots, potatoes are used to thicken soups.

TYPES OF SOUPS

1. **DESSERT SOUP**: Includes vegetables, beans, tubers, tara, etc.
2. **FRUIT SOUP**: Fruit is the primary ingredient and may be served warm or cold depending on the recipe.
3. **COLD SOUP**: May be sweet or savory. The temperature when served is kept at or below room temperature.
4. **ASIAN SOUP** uses tofu.
5. **AFRICAN SOUPS** Egusi soup from Nigeria, Nkatenkwan a heavily spiced soup from Ghana based on groundnut with meat, most often chicken and vegetable added.

BEVERAGES

A beverage is a drink other than water. Beverages are liquids prepared for human consumption. They are portable drinks which have thirst-quenching, stimulating, and nourishing qualities.

CLASSES OF BEVERAGES

- Alcoholic beverages:
- Fermented (beers and wines), distilled (whiskey, spirit liquors)
- Compound distilled beverages
- Brandies and liqueurs
- Bitters, cocktails, eggnog, cider, hard soda, egg flip, punch
- Non-alcoholic beverages: smoothies, milkshakes, tisanes, and cold drinks.

ALCOHOLIC BEVERAGES: These are beverages that contain ethanol

1. ***FERMENTED ALCOHOLIC BEVERAGES:*** These are brewed from fermented cereal mash.

   A. **BEER:** It is brewed from barley, hops and stabilizers. They have a bitter taste. They are fermented malt beverages brewed in different ways. The ideal temperature for serving beer is 40°F.

TYPES OF BEER

- **ALE:** It is a type of beer with a bittering agent. It tastes more strongly of hops than beer. It is brewed using warm fermentation method resulting in a sweet, full- bodied and fruity taste.
- **LAGER:** Beer that is fermented and stored (lagered) in caves for weeks or months at temperatures of about 40$^{OF.}$
- STOUT: It is a dark beer made using roasted malt or roasted barley, hops, water, and yeast. It is stronger and and colored.

B. **WINE**: Wine is a partial or total fermentation of freshly pressed grapes. Berries, apples, cherries, dandelions, elder-berries, palm, honey, or rice can be fermented.

Popular types of wines are table wines, sangria, sparkling wine, champagne, port, sherry, vermouth, and fortified wine.

TYPES OF WINE

- **TABLE WINES**: These are natural wines served with meals. They have an alcoholic content of 10-14o/o. The table wines are dry red wines, dry white wines and rose wines such as Anjou.
- **DESSERT WINES**: they are sweet, still or fortified. The wines that have spirits added to them, often brandy to bring the alcoholic content up to 20% are especially compactible with dessert. The best known of the dessert wine is sherry.
- **CHAMPAGNE**: it is a white wine made from a blend of two types of grapes of pinot noir grapes and pinot chardonnay grapes also known as white grapes. Champagne is fermented twice, once before bottling and once after bottling. Light champagne is obtained when the white grapes are used. Champagne may be dry or sweet depending on the sweetening added after the first fermentation champagne is the only wine that can be served at any time of the day, and any course of a meal. The sweeter champagnes however are more suited for dessert.
- **OTHER SPARKLING WINES**: Burgundy i.e., Anjou rose.
- **COOKING WINES**: The cooking wines are "salted" so that they wouldn't be drunk. It is pointless buying them because the best wines to cook with are drinking wines except the very expensive ones.

2. **DISTILLED BEVERAGES (WHISKIES AND SPIRIT LIQUORS)**: All whiskies are liquors. Distillation is from fermented feed stock such as fruits, vegetables, and cereal grains.

- **WHISKEY**: Is distilled from fermented grain mash such as rye, barley, wheat, maize, malted barley, and malted rye, and aged in wooden casks, generally oak. Distilled beverages such as liquors are called spirits. They are beverages low in sugars and containing at least 35% ABV. Liquors are an alcoholic drink of distilled spirit having 55% ABV. Liquor is the name of liqueur in the U.S.A and Canada. Whiskey is the common spelling while whisky is the British spelling used for Scotch and Canadian whisky.

POPULAR TYPES OF LIQUORS OR SPIRITS

- **GIN**: It is distilled gin made by redistilling white grain spirit which has been flavored with juniper berries. It is neutral grain spirits, crisp, colorless and lightly flavored with juniper berries. Compound gin is made by flavoring neutral grain spirit with juniper berries without redistilling and can be considered flavored vodka. The most common style of gin typically used for mixed drinks is London dry gin.

- **RUM**: This is liquor distilled from sugar syrup or molasses. It is made primarily in the Caribbean. It can be light or soft, can be full-bodied. Light rum is used in cocktails and golden rums in cooking and cocktails.
- **SNAPS OR SCHNAPPS**: The word means any strong dry or colorless liquor in Holland and Germany such as gin in Finland Vodka.
- **SCOTCH**: This is a well-aged blend of grain and malt whiskies made in Scotland.
- **VODKA**: It is highly distilled charcoal filtered colorless liquor distilled from fermented grain mash, or potatoes or sugar beet molasses. Vodka is flavorless and odorless. Has alcohol content of 35o/o to 50o/o ABV. It's a Russian delight. They are usually served after meals or used in mixing drinks.
- **SAKE**: Japanese wine made from rice.

3. ***COMPOUD BEVERAGES (BRANDY AND LIQUEUR)***: Distilled beverages have added flavorings and high sugar content.

- **BRANDY**: This is a distilled wine or fermented fruit juice, well-aged, usually in wood. Has a 40%-60% ethyl ABV. Made from wine grapes, pomace colored with caramel. COGNAC is brandy made in Cognac, France. It is one of the choicest.

- **LIQUEUR** (Cordials and Schnapps in the U.S.A) is a strong alcoholic beverage made from distilled spirits that has been flavored with fruit cream, herbs, spices, flowers, seeds, nut, roots, and barks with added sugar or other sweeteners, sweet and syrupy in consistency and drunk after meals. It has 15% to 30% ABV. The name depends on the flavoring agents used. Categories are fruit, cream, coffee, chocolate, schnapps, and brandy, and anise, nut flavored, and herbal.

4. ***BITTERS:*** Bitters are used in making cocktails, taken as aperitifs, liqueurs, and medicine. Many bitters are said to be good for digestion. They are made of aromatic seeds, herbs, barks, and plants from carefully guarded recipes. All are bitter or bittersweet and many have a high alcoholic content

TYPES OF BITTERS

- **COMPARI**: This is Italy's most popular bitters. It is usually mixed with soda when drinking.

- **ANGOSTURA**: This is the best known of all the bitters, created by a German doctor in Trinidad.

5. ***COCKTAILS***: A cocktail is any beverage that contains three or more ingredients, one of these at least must be alcohol. It is an alcoholic drink mixed with two or more ingredients at least one alcoholic component which can be a distilled spirit, beer, or wine, one sweet component and a souring or bittering ingredient mixed with other ingredients such as fruits juice or cream.

6. ***EGGNOG***: This is a drink consisting of rum, brandy, vodka, whisky, bourbon or other alcohol or a combination of liquors mixed with whisk eggs, milk, and sugar. It is usually garnished with ground cinnamon or nutmeg. Traditional egg nog is made with sugar, raw eggs, spices, nutmeg, cream, chocolate curls as toppings. Eggnog is sometimes called egg milk punch.

7. ***CIDER***: (Apple juice or apple wine): This is fermented alcohol with 1.2% to 8.5% ABV.

8. ***HARD SODA***: It is manufactured in the style of a soft drink.

9. ***EGG FLIP:*** This is an alcoholic drink made from egg, sugar and brandy or sherry.

10. ***PUNCH***: A beverage of fruit juice and sometimes a soft drink or carbonated water, often spiced and mixed with a wine or a liquor base.

HOW TO SERVE WINE

1. Red wine should be served at room temperature

2. White and rose wines should be chilled before serving about 40-45°, about 2 to 3 hours in the refrigerator

3. Champagne should be well chilled so with sparkling burgundy. Red wines should be uncorked about an hour before serving so that they have a chance to "breathe" and develop full flavor.

TYPES OF GLASSWARE

Many standard and patterns and sizes of glassware are available to serve each drink. Most glass drinking vessels are either tumblers, flat-bottom glasses with no handle, foot, or stem, or stemware which has a bowl on a stem above a flat base. Neither a tumbler, footed, nor a stem, yard (beer) is a very tall, conical beer glass, with a round ball base, usually hung on the wall when empty.

COLLINS GLASSWARE: A Collins glass is a glass tumbler, holding 240-350ml, used to serve mixed drink, named after Tom Collins. This glass is somewhat narrower and holds less than the similar highball glass.

HIGHBALL GLASS: A highball glass is a glass, holding 240-350ml used to serve a mixed drink, or highball. This glass is taller than an Old-Fashioned glass, and shorter than a Collins glass.

SHOT GLASS: It is a small glass used for measuring or serving up to 94ml of liquor. Modern shot glass holds a thicker base and sides than the whisky glass.

PINT GLASS: A pint glass is a drinking vessel holding an imperial pint (568ml) of liquid and is usually used for beer. Three common shapes of pint glass are found (conical, jug, and flared top), though others are available. Pints are considered good for serving stouts, porters, and English ales.

PILSNER GLASS: A pilsner glass is a glass used to serve many types of light beers, but is intended for its namesake, the pilsner. Pilsner glasses are smaller than a pint glass, usually in 250ml or 330ml sizes. They are tall, slender, and tempered. Wheat beer glasses are often mistakenly referred to as pilsner glasses, but a true pilsner glass has an even taper without a curvature. Pilsner glasses are made to showcase the color, effervescence, and clarity of the pilsner, as well as to maintain a nice head.

FLUTE GLASS: A flute glass is the preferred serving vessel for Belgian lagers and fruit beers. The narrow shape helps maintain carbonation, while providing a strong aromatic front. Flute glasses display the lively carbonation, sparkling color, and soft lacing of this distinct style.

GOBLET OR CHALICE: Chalices and goblets are large, stemmed, bowl-shaped glasses adequate for serving heavy Belgian ales, German bocks, and other big sipping beers. The different between goblet and chalice is typically in the glass thickness. Goblets tend to be more delicate and thinner, while the chalice is heavy and thick-walled.

SNIFTERS: Typically use for serving brandy or cognac, a snifter is ideal for capturing the volatiles of aromatic beers, such as Belgian ales, India pale ales, Barley wines and wheat wines. The shape helps trap the volatiles, while allowing swirling to agitate them and produce an intense aroma.

WHEAT BEER GLASS: A wheat beer glass is a glass used to serve wheat beer, known as Weizenbier or Weibbier. The German glass generally holds 500ml with room for foam or "head". It is much taller than a pint glass. It is very narrow at the bottom and slightly wider at the top. In other countries such as Belgian, the glass may hold 250ml or 330ml. The tall glass provides room for the often thick, fluffy heads produced by the style which traps aromas and is visually pleasing.

TULIP GLASS: A tulip glass not only helps trap the aroma, but also aids in maintaining large heads, creating a visual and olfactory sensation. The body is bulbous, but the top flares out to form a lip which helps head retention. It is recommended for serving Scottish ales, barley wines, Belgian ales, and other aromatic beers.

COCTAIL GLASS: A cocktail glass or champagne glass, or stem cocktail glass, is a drinking glass with a cone-shaped bowl (the tip of the cone forming approximately a 90-degree angle in the cross section) on a stem above a flat base, used to serve a cocktail or champagne. As with other stem wear the stem allows the drinker to hold the glass without affecting the temperature of the drink. One variation is the double martini glass which is taller and wider at the opening than a standard martini glass.

RED WINE GLASS: Glasses for red wine are characterized by their rounder, wider bowl, which gives the wine a chance to breathe. Since most reds are meant to be consumed at room temperature, the wider the bowl also allows the wine to cull more quickly after hand contact has warmed it. Red wine glasses can have particular styles of their own, such as as:

Bordeaux glass: Tall with a wide bowl and is designed for full bodied red wines like Cabernet and Merlot as it directs the wine to the back of the mouth.

Burgundy glass: Larger than the Bordeaux glass, it has a larger bowl to accumulate aromas of more delicate red wines such as Pinot Noir. This style of glass directs wine to the tip of the tongue.

WHITE WINE: White wine glasses are generally narrower although not as narrow as champagne flutes, with somewhat straight or tulip-shaped sides. The narrowness of the white wine glass allows the chilled to retain its temperature for two reasons:

1. The reduced surface of the glass (in comparison to red wine glasses) means less circulation around the glass and warming the glass.
2. The smaller bowl of the glass means less contact between the hand and the glass, and so body heat does not transfer as easily or as fast to the wine.

CHAMPAGNE FLUTE: Champagne flutes are characterized by a long stem with a tall narrow bowl on top. The shape is designed to keep sparkling wine attractive and inviting during its consumption. The glass is designed to be held by the stem to prevent the heat from the hand warming up the champagne. The bowl itself is designed in a manner to help retain the signature carbonation in the beverage. This is achieved by reducing the surface area at the opening of the bowl. Champagne flutes are often used at formal engagements such as award ceremonies and weddings.

SHERRY GLASS: A narrow glass is a drink wear generally used for serving aromatic alcoholic beverages, such as sherry, port, aperitifs, and liqueurs, and layered shooters. An ISO-standard size sherry glass is 120ml. The copita, with its aroma-enhancing narrow taper, is a type of sherry glass.

COUPETTE GLASS: A modified version of the cocktail glass. Used for serving drinks where the rim of the glass is required to be coated in either sugar or salt or any other condiments used to make some of the more exotic drinks such as margaritas.

PILCHER: This larger container usually has a handle and a lip or spout for pouring the contents into several glasses. Available in glass or plastic. Generally used for serving beer for keg for draft beer.

OLD FASHIONED GLASS: The old-fashioned glass, rocks glass, or "low-ball" is a short tumbler used for serving liquor "on the rocks" meaning over ice, or cocktails having few ingredients. It is named after the old-fashioned cocktail, traditionally served in such a glass. A White Russian is traditionally served in the the Fashioned Glass.

YARD GLASS: A yard (or yard glass) is a very tall glass used for drinking beer; a yard or (or yard of ale) also (variable) quantity of beer held by such a glass. The glass is approximate (hence the name) and holds 2 imperial pints (1.14 liters) of liquid. The glass is shaped with a bulb at the bottom and widening shaft which constitutes most of the height. Because the glass is so long and, in any case, does not have a stable flat base, it is hung on the wall when not in use.

COFFEE- MUG: Almost a smaller version of the beer mug made of thick heavy glass and used for coffee.

IRISH COFFEE CUP: A uniquely shaped glass with a handle that is used to serve any hot beverage such as Spanish coffee or cocoa.

HANDLING OF GLASSWARE

1. Glassware is highly fragile and almost delicate and expensive: hence almost care has to be taken while handling glass equipment.
2. Glasses are normally stored in a glass pantry and should be places upside down in single rows on paper-lined shelves, to prevent dust settling in them.
3. Tumblers should not be stacked onside one another as this may result in heavy breakages and accidents.
4. The appearance of the drink depends on the glass therefore, the glass should be sparkling clean and attractive in shape and style.
5. When glassware is machine or handwashed, each individual item must be polished and dried with a glass linen, as water leaves stains on the glasses.
6. Glasses whether clean or dirty have to be handled by the base or stem, since the fingerprints left on the glass necessitating polishing.

POPULAR SIZES OF STEMWEAR AND GLASSWEAR

A. 234 ml- Old-fashioned cocktail, B. 375 ml- double old-fashioned or other tall drinks, C. 375 ml Highball, D. 281 ml. Scotch and Soda, E. 187 whisky sour or other short cocktail, F. 46.8 ml jigger (whiskey), G. 321 ml all-purpose goblet, H. 281 sherbet and wine glass, I. 218 to 250ml low sherbet and wine glass, J. 188 ml whiskey sour glass, K. 125 ml cocktail glass, L. 188 ml claret glass, M. 125 ml wine (white) or burgundy glass, N. 31 ml cordial for liqueurs, O. 141 ml sherry glass, P. 469ml. Luncheon goblet.

Q. 188 ml orange juice or liqueur glass.

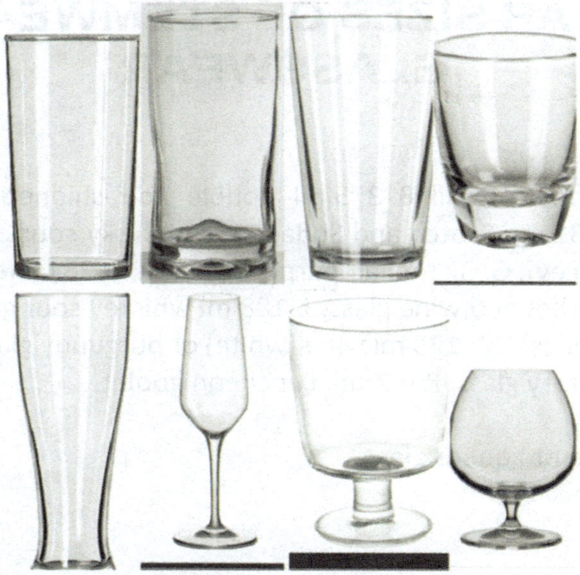

Top (LR) Collins, highball, pint glass, shot. Bottom (LR) Pilsner, flute, goblet or chalice, snifters

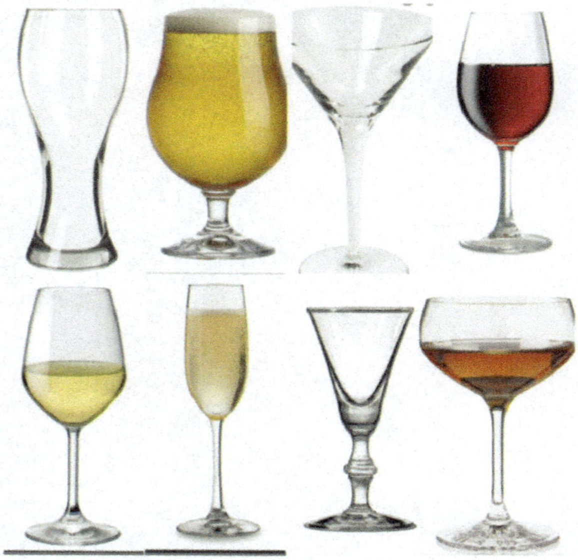

Top (LR) Wheat beer glass, tulip, cocktail glass, red wine glass. Bottom (LR) White wine glass, champagne glass, sherry glass, coupet

NON-ALCOHOLIC BEVERAGES

1. ***SMOOTHIES:*** It is a creamy beverage made of fresh fruit blended with juice, yogurt, honey or syrup, chocolate, and peanut butter.

2. ***MILK SHAKES (THICK SHAKE, THICK MILKSHAKE, and FRAPPÉ):*** It is a cold drink made of milk, a sweet flavoring such as fruit syrup, chocolate sauce and typically ice cream whisk until frothy

3. ***TISANES:*** Are mostly plant products. They have soothing effects, digestive effects; can be sed as aperitifs and as diuretics. Lemon grass is a tisane. It is sometimes called fever grass, barbed wire grass, silky heads, or citronella grass.

4. ***COLD DRINKS AND TYPES:*** (aerated drinks, spring water/mineral water, squash, juices, and syrups)
    - **AERATED-DRINKS** are charged or aerated with carbon gas. Examples are soda water, dry ginger, fizzy lemonade, ginger beer, Coca-Cola, Pepsi, and others.
    - **SPRING WATER/ MINERAL WATER**
    - **SQUASH**: It is a highly sweetened (often fruit based) concentrate, which is diluted with a liquid, most commonly water before drinking. Squash is created by mixing one part concentrate with four or five parts of water (depending on concentration and personal taste) directly into a mug, or glass, or into a jug. Squashes are also mixed with spirits or cocktails. The most common flavors are orange, apple and black currants, lemon, peppermint, mixed fruit, summer fruits and lemon-lime. Other flavors include peach, strawberry, passion fruit, custard apple and kiwi fruit.
    - **JUICE:** It is prepared by mechanically squeezing or macerating fresh fruits or vegetables without the application of heat or solvent. Popular juices are apple, orange, prune, lemon, grapefruit, cherry, pineapple, tomato, carrot, grape, strawberry, cranberry, pomegranate, guava, sapota, celery. A variety of fruits can be combined into single juice drinks. Popular blends are cran-apple (cranberry and apple) and apple and blackcurrant. Juices are used for cocktails and mixed with spirits.
    - **SYRUP**: It is a thick, viscous liquid, containing a large number of dissolved sugars (60 to 65% brix), but showing little tendency for crystallization of dissolved sugar as a long drink. Some examples of syrup are: Orgeat (almond), Cassis (black currant), Citronelle (lemon), Framboise (raspberry), and Cerise (cherry).

5. ***HOT BEVERAGES: (Tea, Coffee, Cocoa)***
   TEA: One of the most widely consumed stimulant beverages in the morning. It is the most popular non-alcoholic beverage.

Types of tea

- **Black tea:** (English breakfast and Darjecling)
- **Green tea**: (It is not fermented)
- **Oolong tea:** Cross between black and green tea in color and taste.
- **White tea:** The least processed. It is not oxidized or rolled but simply withered and presented in a variety of ways such as follows: Drip brewed and Percolated

FRENCH-PRESSED/CAFTIÈRE COFFEE: May be served with no additives (black coffee).

COCOA: It is a powder made from cacao seeds (bean) after fermentation, roasting, shelled, ground and freed from most of their fat.

ADVANTAGES OF BEVERAGES

REFRESHMENT: used to relieve thirst. Non-alcoholic beverage such as plain or carbonated water, lime juice, ginger ale, and other bottled beverages, fruit juices, and iced tea or coffee are refreshing drinks and are used to relieve thirst.

NOURISHMENT: pasteurized milk, butter milk, chocolate and cocoa drinks, eggnog made with rum, fruit juices, glucose water, and lemonade provide nutrients and help in nourishing the body.

STIMULANT: tea coffee, cocoa, chocolate beverages help in stimulating the system.

SOOTHING AGENT: warm milk and hot tea have a soothing effect and are used for this purpose.

APPETIZERS: soups, fruit juice and alcoholic drinks in limited quantities increase an individual's appetite and thereby food consumption.

ENTERTAINMENT: in social occasions.

CAMEROON TRADITIONAL ALCOHOLIC DRINKS

(Shaah, kwacha, Bili-Bili, Afofo (Quoh in Tikar) which is a distilled drink, and palm wine)

The Cameroonian brewed drinks are done mostly by women. The shaah, kwacha, Bili-Bili are the famous ones known. The shaah and kwacha are brewed from corn while Bili-Bili is from millet. The production methods are similar, which include steeping of the raw product, grinding, fermentation, and sieving. These drinks have brought a lot of economic power to the women, who have used the income to educate their children. The palm wine is a natural drink, being a specialty of men. Women raise money with the production of the foléré drink, a drink of the Sorrel leaves.

THE SHAAH

Shaah is a famous drink brewed from fermented corn. It is a product of Donga-Mantung Division, Bui Division, Ngoketungia Division and Menchum Division of the North West Region of Cameroon. It is brewed by women which has brought economic power to the rural women of these divisions. Shaah is drunk from calabashes which keep it cool.

KWACHA

Kwacha or kwata is brewed almost the same way as the shaah, but for the second fermentation which the shaah does not have. It is a heavier drink than shaah. It is also brewed by women.

PALM WINE

This a natural drink found in Cameroon and some West African countries. In Cameroon it is commonly called white mimbo, palmwine, matango and sometimes called Bamboo milk. This drink is a whitish sap which comes from a variety of palm trees. The palm wine is from an unbranched evergreen tree with very long feathered or fan-shaped leaves. The raffia palm wine is extracted from another variety of palm tree which has a short trunk and very long leaves. The "MBUH" wine is from a variety of the raffia palm which has very long and healthy bamboos. The raffia and palm wines have many names such as "Mulluh" in Mezam Division in the North West Region, "Ndunkue or Ndu nkua in the Bamileke dialects of the West Region.

Palm wine is consumed in the southern part of Cameroon when people are assembled for special occasions. In the North West Region, Ndop in Ngoketungia Division, and Bafut in Mezam Division produce good quality palmwine while Mankon also in Mezam Division is noted for the best raffia wine. Batibo in Momo Division, also of the North West region is the greatest producer of Mbuh raffia palm wine.

Raffia wine of good quality is also produced in Babajou in the Bamboutous Division of the West region and in Noun Division of the West Regions called Bamoun raffia wine. Certain herbs are introduced into the Bamoun palms to activate the flow of the sap. In the Centre and South Regions of Cameroon palm wine is also collected from the palm trees.

The first collection of palm wine or raffia wine is usually very sweet and afterward becomes strong that means alcoholic. The older palms produce more sap than the young ones. Once the raffia starts producing wine it can continue for about 1 to 1½ months before it dries off. The wine is collected in calabashes and sometimes in plastic bottles.

PARTY AND SPECIAL OCCASION DISHES

Cameroonians are a very hospitable people, who serve food and drinks when visited at home or when there are special occasions. Where two or three are gathered, food is served. Cameroonians are party loving people. Cocktail parties are not common because they are considered light and not filling. The parties usually have finger foods called chewable, served in addition to heavy foods. These chewable are served in almost all parties; be it funerals, weddings, or anniversaries. They take the place of hors d'oeuvres before the main dishes. They maybe savory or sweet such as cakes, chin chin, puff balls, fried fish, fried chicken, fish rolls, or pot roast groundnuts. Desserts are usually not part of a traditional Cameroonian meal, for sweet dishes can be served as aperitifs, first courses, or hors d'oeuves. As regards to snacks, Cameroonians love to snack because of the long duration out of home. Fruits are favorite snacks. Vegetables such as carrots are also a favorite snack. Nuts and fresh roast or cooked, corn on the cob is seasonal snacks.

To celebrate the birth of a baby, usually called "Born House", the main dish is pottage plantain called "pickin plantain". It is cooked with heavy chunks of meat, bitter leaves, and a lot of palm oil. "Born house" plantain is served with other dishes depending on the host, which usually includes the dish of the host's region origin.

A lot of money is spent on food during funerals. There is the wake keep, the actual burial day, and the days after burial when guests and family members have to be fed. Funeral foods are usually heavy foods such as pottage plantains, corn fufu and njama- njama, Jollof rice, water fufu and eru soup.

In addition to the above in the North West region of Cameroon, boiled groundnuts/ shelled corn, cooked fresh corn on cob, dried cooked corn on cob and fresh boiled groundnuts are served. A recent innovation is the introduction of sandwiches, fish rolls, and scotch eggs, and fish pies served at these occasions. Beans koki is a favorite because it serves the host the hazel of providing serving utensils like plates. During these funerals, meat is a very important aspect. Chicken, pigs, goats, and cattle are slaughtered. Once this is done there is hope that the guests will be well fed.

COCKTAIL PARTY DISHES (FINGER FOODS)

Chin-chin, fish rolls, meat rolls, scotch eggs, meat balls, banana akra, beans akra, cakes, sandwiches, beef soya, sardine rolls, puff balls beans koki, fruit kebabs, chips (plantains, Irish, potatoes), caramels (groundnuts, coconuts), mandasi, sombasa, fried fish, fried chicken, fried meat, stuffed eggs, mbon-lep, masoma, egusi pudding, pili-pili viande, pilig-pili poison, croquette de farine, gateau au mais, and gateau au yaourt.

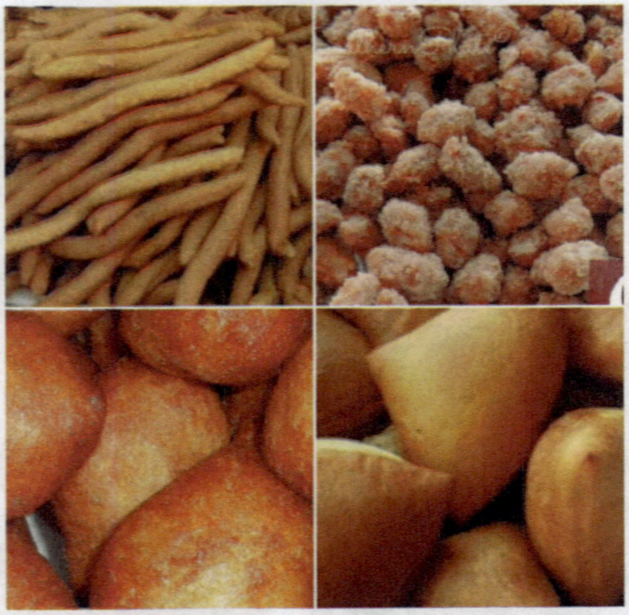

Kurukuru (groundnut/corn paste), sugared groundnuts (groundnut sweets), puff-puff, mandasi.

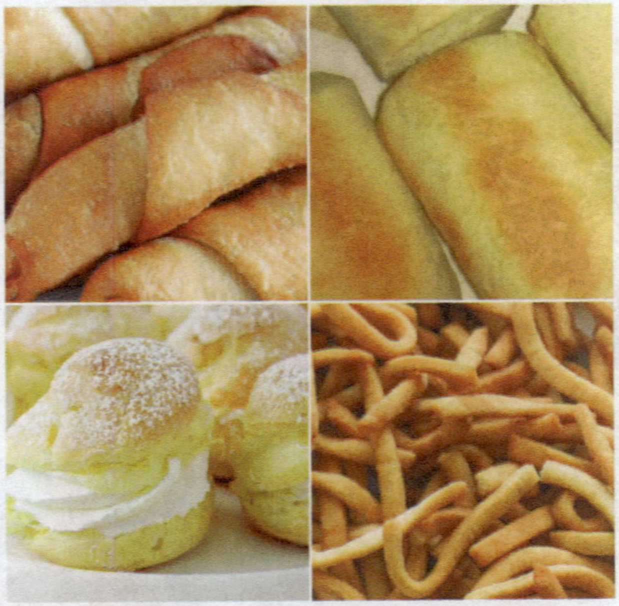

Fried fish roll, baked fish roll, cream puffs, chin-chin (Immaculate bites?

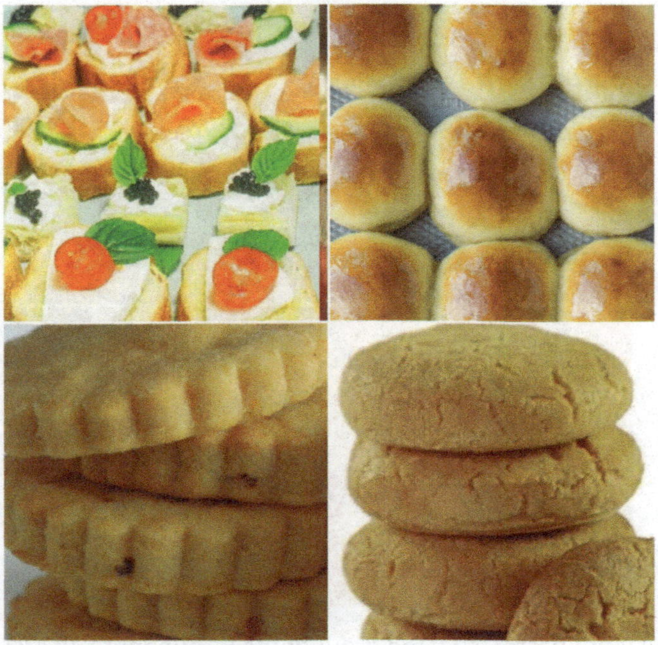

Canapés, Ardith's rolls, Shrewsbury biscuits, savoury biscuits.

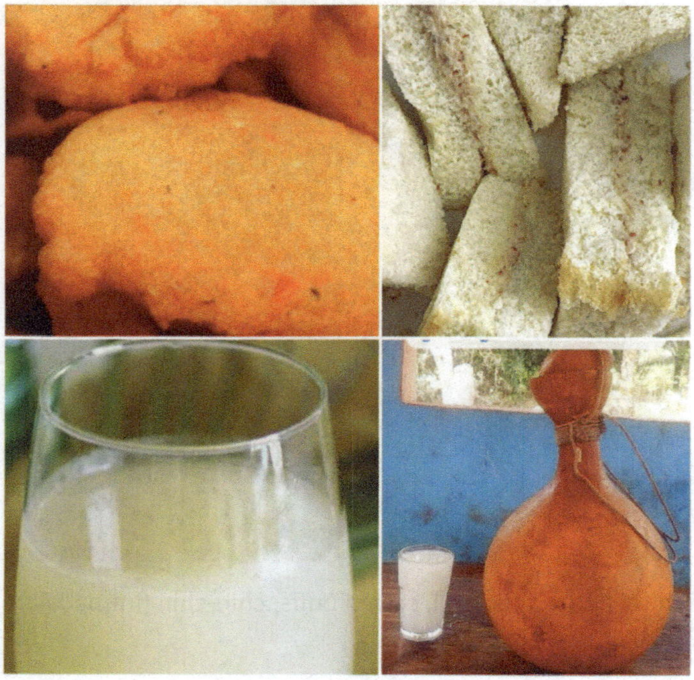

Beans Akra, simple sandwich, palm wine, palmwine Calabash (gourd)

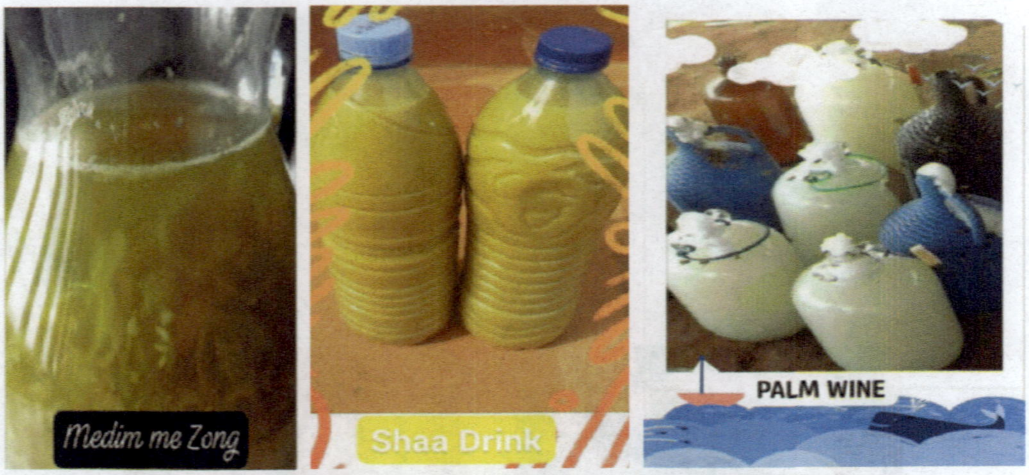

Medim me Zong Shaa drink and Palm wine

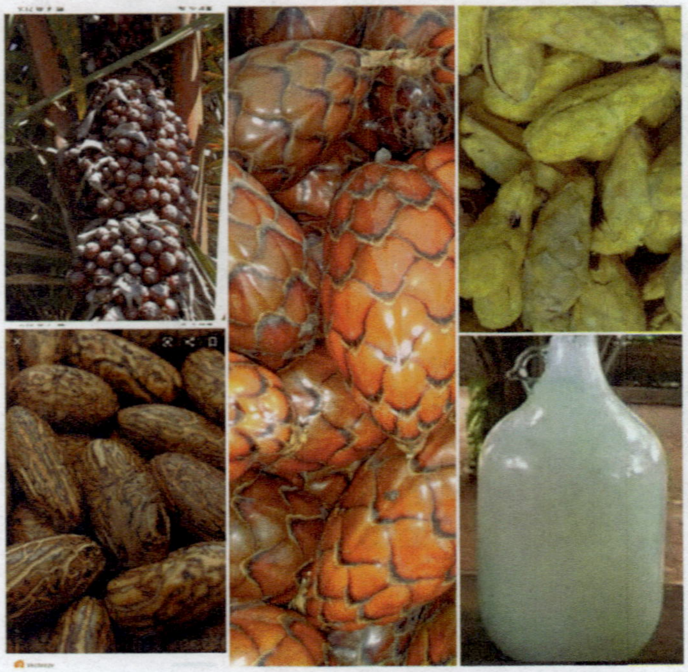

Raffia Raffia palm fruit, prepared fruit in yellow (akob), seed from akob, raffia palm wine

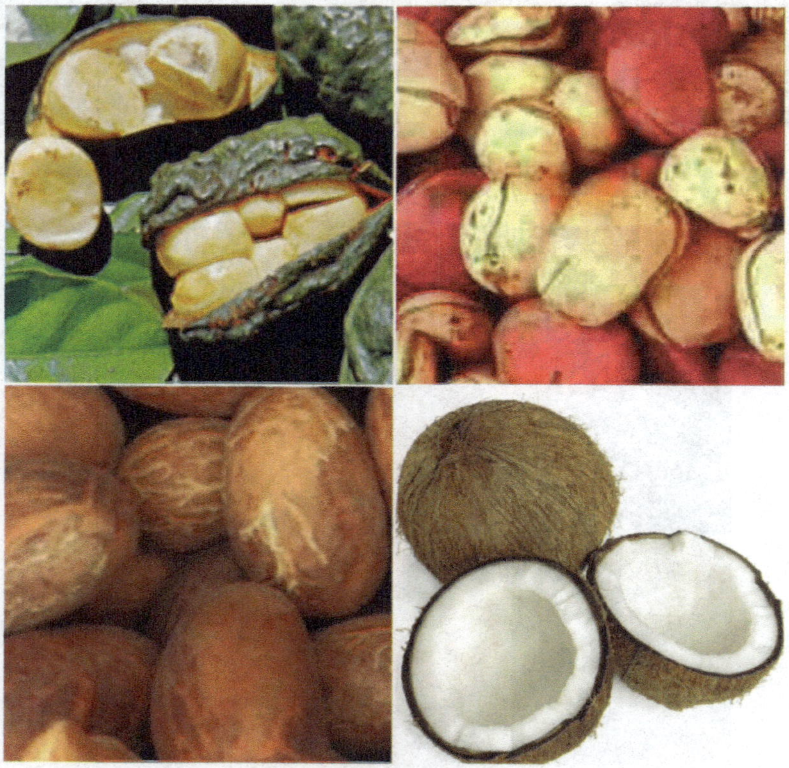

Colanut, bitter kola, coconut.

CUSTARD

Custard is a variety of culinary preparations based on a cooked mixture of milk and/or cream and egg yolk. Depending on how much egg or thickener is used custard may vary in consistency from a thin pouring sauce (crème Anglaise) to a thick pastry cream (crème patisserie). Most common custards are used as dessert sauces or desserts and typically include sugar and vanilla. Custard (crème moulée) refers to only egg-thickened custard. Pastry cream (crème patissière) or confectioners' custard) refers to custard when starch is added. Custard is called crème in French

VARIATIONS OF CUSTARD

CUSTARD (CRÈME OU CRÈME MOULÉE): egg-thickened custard.

CONFECTIONNERS' CUSTARD (CRÈME PATISSIÈRE): combination of milk or cream, egg yolks, fine sugar, flour or some other starch, and usually a flavoring such as vanilla, chocolate, or lemon is added. It is also called pastry cream.

CRÈME ANGLAISE: Egg is used alone as a thickener.

CRÈME ANGLAISE COLLÉE: When gelation is added

BLANCMANGE: When the custard is thickened with starch (without eggs). After the custard is thickened, it may be mixed with other ingredients.

CHIBOUST CREAM: Mixed with egg whites and gelatin.

CRÈME LÉGÈRE: custard mixed with whipped cream.

CRÈME MOUSSELINE (German buttercream) beating in soften butter.

QUICHE is a savory custard tard.

TIMBALE: (vegetable loaf) made of custard base mixed with chopped savory ingredients.

CUSTARD ROYALE: A thick custard cut into decorative shapes and used to garnish soup, stew, or broth.

TYPES OF CUSTARDS
(STOVE TOP)
(STIRRED CUSTARDS)

They are also known as soft custard, custard sauce or boiled custard.

They are stirred while being cooked over low heat or in a double boiler to a smooth, creamy, and thickened fluid consistency.

BAVARIAN CREAM: A cold dessert composed of a cooked, richer custard, whipped cream, various flavorings, such as fruit purée. Chocolate, liqueurs, stabilized with gelatin. The mixture may be spooned into stemmed glasses or into a decorative mold to be unmolded when set.

CHARLOTTE: A classic molded dessert. The mold lined with sponge cake, lady fingers or buttered bread. The traditional mold is pail-shaped, but any mold can be used. The lined mold is filled with layers (or mixture) of fruit and cooked custard or whipped cream that has been fortified with gelatin. The dessert is thoroughly chilled and unmolded before serving.

CHARLOTTE RUSSE: Is a lady finger shell filled with ethereal Bavarian cream and decorated elaborately with whipped-cream rosettes. The classic apple charlotte is a buttered-bread shell filled with spiced, sautéed apples. Unlike other charlottes, this one is baked and served hot.

CITRUS (LEMON) CURDS: A custard made with lemon juice, butter, sugar, and eggs and used as a spread or filling. But curds can be made in other flavors, such as raspberry, lime and orange for example.

CREAM PIES: The filling is made from a cooked custard or mousse, spread in a cooled pre-baked pie shell versus a baked custard pie when the filling, uncooked custard is poured into a pie shell and both are baked together. A pumpkin pie is considered to be a custard pie as a pecan pie.

CRÈME ANGLAISE: (VANILLA SAUCE): The French term for a rich custard sauce that can be served hot or cold over cake, fruit, or other desserts. It is also called custard sauce,

English cream and known as "Mother sauce" in pastry. It is used as base in many creams, mousses, ice cream and desserts. It is based on milk sugar and egg yolks.

PASTRY CREAM: It is considered the "Mother of all creams" classic stovetop custard made with starch, such as corn starch. It is simply heated and stirred directly on the stove until boiling. It is then strained before cooling (crème pâtissier)

VANILLA SAUCE: considered a "mother sauce in pastry.

BAKED CUSTARDS

They are not stirred during the baking process, thus giving a more solid texture. The use of water bath helps heat sensitive egg custards bake low and slow in the oven, protecting the delicate egg proteins.

SIMPLE BAKED CUSTARD: Are the lightest of all of the custard desserts. They have a lower ratio of eggs to liquid (typically milk) and as a result, will gel with little structure and cannot be unmolded before serving.

CHEESECAKES: Sometimes classified as a flourless cake, it is basically a custard baked in the oven, however it can also be unbaked or typically molded in a dessert ring or spring form pan then simply chilled before unmolding.

CRÈME BRULÉE: It's French for burnt custard in the oven and served in its same container. It is a creamy and sinfully rich dessert, which blends the cool velvet smoothness of custard topped with a crisp, caramelized layer of sugar, caramelized just before serving. Recipes usually contain heavy cream and lots of egg yolks.

CRÈME CARAMEL: Is fairly light custard, often made with milk as all or part of the dairy and with added yolks for some degree of richness, baked in a ramekin or mold with a layer of caramel at the bottom. It is unmolded before serving, and the caramel pulls around the custard. In French it is known as crème Renversée. Examples are **Custard Pie**: Is when the filling, uncooked custard is poured into a pie shell and both are baked together.

FLAN: Spanish or Mexican version of crème caramel, but usually richer and denser than crème caramel because recipes contain more eggs and yolks, some cream or evaporated or condensed milk. It is also baked in a caramel-lined mold. When inverted, the caramel baked on the bottom becomes the topping.

POTS DE CRÈME: French for "pot of cream" is traditionally served in small, lidded porcelain cups and a rich custards dessert, relatives of crème Brulée, crème caramel, and flan. This custard is very rich, like crème brulée because recipes use a very high proportion of egg yolks to whole eggs, if used at all.

PUDDING CAKES: They are basically baked egg custards.

SAVOURY

A savory is a savory item served on varying shapes of toast; in tartelette (round), and baguettes (oval); in bouchees, flan rings or as an omelet or soufflé. Savory food has a salty or spicy flavor rather than a sweet one. Savory dishes can be served hot, cold, warm, at room temperature or chilled. They can be spicy, mild flavored or plain.

On the lunch and dinner menu, the savory is generally served as an alternative to a sweet, whilst in a banquet it may be a course on its own, coming between the entremets (sweet) and the dessert (fresh fruits and nuts). In la carte menu, the savories are listed in a section of their own.

SAVOURIES

The term savories covers a range of items served either as Savory course (served as a traditional meal where the item is highly tangy and refreshes the palate after the sweet and prior to the serious business of the dinner drinks), Cocktail savories (these are mainly of various canapés and are eaten as appetizers served with drinks prior to meal, during a cocktail party), Sandwiches (these are sometimes categorized as savories particularly sandwiches), or small items (are eaten as snacks in bars, coffee shops and cafes.

TYPES OF SAVOURY

There are eight main types of savory:

1. Savory using a sauce: These are usually “salpicon” based using béchamel sauce, curry sauce, and devil sauce, 2. Grilled items, 3. Shallow fried items. 4 shallow poached items. 5. Scrambled eggs. 6. Short pastry items, 7. Savory soufflés. 8. Puff pastry items.

SAVOURY DISHES

The following are the popular savory dishes:

1. ***SAVOVRY ON TOAST***

Welsh rabbit, rarebit, or welsh rarebit: is traditionally a sauce made with a mixture of cheese and butter poured over toasted bread which has been buttered. In current popular use, cheese on toast is simply slices of cheese placed on toasted bread and melted by heat from above in a grill or salamander.

- **Buck Rabbit**: A welsh rarebit garnished with garnished with a poached egg.
- **Moelle on Toast:** Chilled marrow is sliced and poached gently in a little white stock. Drained well and dressed on hot buttered toast. Easoned and coated with beurre, noisette, sprinkled with chopped parsley.
- **Haddock on toast:** Poached haddock and flake mixed with cream sauce. Spread on toast and decorated to serve.
- **Anchovies on toast**: Breads are toasted, and anchovy's fillets are laid side by side. Finished with the heated oil from the anchovies. Decorated with sieved hard-boiled yolk of egg and chopped parsley.
- **Sardines on toast:** Sardines are split, and backbone is removed from head to tail is laid on the toast, and finished with the oil from the sardine.
- **Roes on toast:** Roes are shallow fried and dresses on toast. Sprinkled with lemon juice coated with beurre noisette and served.

2. CANAPES: Generally, canapés are small, decorative pieces of bread toasted or untoasted) that are topped with a savory garnish such as anchovy, cheese, or some type of bread.

- **Canape Baron:** Garnished with slices of fried mushrooms, grilled bacon, and poached bone marrow.
- **Canape Ritchie:** Creamed haddock, garnished with slices of hard-boiled eggs.
- **Canape Quo Vadis:** Grilled roes garnished with small mush room heads.
- **Canape Nina:** half small grilled tomato, garnished with mushroom head and a pickled walnut.
- **Canape Charlemagne:** Garnish with shrimps bound with a curry sauce.
- **Angels on horseback:** Shucked oysters wrapped in bacon, though sometimes scallops are used in
- place of the oysters. This is then baked in the oven and quite often served on toast.

- **Devils on horseback:** Contains a pitted prune (Dates are sometimes used) stuffed with mango
- chutney and wrapped in bacon. This is then baked in the oven and quite often served on toast, with watercress. Hot pepper sauce is often added.

3. CROUTS: These are shaped pieces of bread approximately ¼ inch thick, shallow fried.

- **Croute derby:** Spread with ham puree and garnished with a pickled walnut.
- **Croute Windsor:** Spread with ham puree and garnished with small grilled mushrooms.
- **Croute Diane:** partly cooked chicken livers (fried) wrapped in streaky bacon and grilled on a skewer.
- **Scotch wookcock:** Scrambled egg garnished with a trellis of anchovy and studded with capes.

4. TARTLETTES: (ROUND) OR BAQUETTES (OVAL): They are normally made from unsweetened short crust pastry.

- **Charles V:** Soft roes mixed with butter, covered with cheese soufflé mixture, and baked in the oven.
- **Favorite**: Filed with cheese soufflé mixture and slices of truffle. Garnished with slices of crayfish tails or prawns.
- **Haddock:** Filled with diced haddock bound with a curry sauce, sprinkled with breadcrumbs and cooked au gratin.

5. BOUCHEES: These are small puff pastry cases. A small edition of a vol-au-vent. They have various fillings: shrimp, lobster, prawn, and haddock.

- **Omelets**: Two / three omelets with various flavors such as mushroom, spinach, sardine, anchovy, haddock, cheeses etc.

6. FLAN: These are made from unsweetened short crust pastry.

- **Quiche Lorraine:** Flan made from unsweetened short crust pastry and filled with rashers of streaky bacon and slices of cheese covered with a savory egg custard mixture and baked in an oven.

7. SOUFFLÉS: These are made in soufflé dishes. Various flavors such as mushrooms, spinach, sardine, anchovy, haddock, cheeses etc. are used.

SERVICE OF SAVOURIES

1. The following cover should be laid for savories: hot fish plate, Side knife, and sweet fork.

2. The accompaniments are to be set as follows: Cayenne pepper, placed on the side plate on table, Cruet, to be replaced if previously removed when clearing the main course, Peppermill, placed on side plate on table, and Worcester sauce, only to offered with a meat savory.

3. If a variety of hot and cold sweets are being ordered by a party of people then the cold items must be served first followed by the hot items. The correct cutlery and flatware are laid before serving and the necessary accompaniments are all on the table before service commences.

CAMEROON FLOUR PROCESSING

CORN FLOUR

Select corn, winnow it to get rid of the loose skin and broken cobs. If corn was treated wash and sun it. Grind in a corn mill. Sun it and put in an airtight container. Sun it frequently to prevent molding.

HAUSA CORN FLOUR

Select corn, winnow it. Soak in water and cover. Let stand for about 2 days. After 2 days drain very well. Grind in a corn meal. Spread in the sun to dry. Sieve and spread again to dry.

Store in an airtight container.

BAMOUN CORN FLOUR

Select corn, winnow it. Peel corn in a peeling/grinding mill
Soak corn for a day. Drain very well, add pieces of shredded dried cassava, grind spread in the sun to dry. Sieve corn flour. Dry again in the sun
Store in an airtight container and use as needed

YAM OR CASSAVA FLOUR

Any quantity of cassava flour
Scrub the cassava very well. Rinse. Slice thinly. Boil water
Spread sliced cassava in a large basket and suspend basket on sticks over a basin.
Pour the boiling water all over the cassava and cover to keep in steam while the water drains. Spread partially cooked cassava into the sun until dry.
Grind in a mill and sieve to get the fine flour. Dry further and store in an air-tight container for use.

NB: Cassava maybe grated, boiled, and squeezed, dried in a basket over fire or in the sun. Store when dry. Grind and sieve dry balls into fine flour when needed. Dried cassava flour is called nkum-nkum or Elubo.

WATER FOOFOO PASTE

Any quantity of cassava (10-20 or more). Peel cassava remove woody and spoiled parts. Cut into 10-12cm length. Wash and remove midrib. Steep cassava in a pot with a lid for 2 to 4 days depending on the climate. Remove from water and grate, wash in a colander. Stand the water and let it settle. Collect the sediment and put in a clean bag. Tie firmly. Press under heavy weights for one day. Remove from bag and store in a refrigerator in a covered container or stand in a covered container with water over it. Use when needed. It will keep for 3 to 4 weeks

RICE FLOUR

3 cups rice will give 4 to 4½ cups flour
Water
Select rice, wash, and allow to steep in water for 30 to 40 minutes. Remove from steeping water and drain. Spread on a tea cloth to dry. When almost dry, grind and sieve to obtain fine flour. Dry flour until perfectly dry. Store in an air-tight container. Use as desired. Yields about 4 to 4½ cups flour.

CASSAVA BATONS OR CHIKWANGUES

(MIONDO AND BOBOLO)

Ingredients

Cassava tubers
Water
Ngongo leaves
Bamboo ropes

Method

Steep the cassava tubers in water for 3 to 5 days. When soft remove the tiny veins from the pulp. Let it ferment for 1 day and allow to drain. Generally, the pulp is tied in jute bags and heavy objects are placed on it to aid drainage. Grind the paste finely (for miondos) and coarsely for bobolo. Wrap in reed leaves and tie with bamboo ropes. For miondo which is a Douala specialty make fine batons or baguette-shapes of about 1cm large by 25cm long. Two of this is jointed to form one. Each of the two is called a **"dibaka"** in the Douala language. The Bobolo or Bebobolo is a Yaounde specialty, about 5cm in diameter and 30cm long. The batons are placed in a steamer with just a little water and steamed.

CAMEROON FLOUR

Flour is processed from the staple foods. They are used in many ways in food preparation.

S/N	ENGLISH NAME	FRENCH NAME	BOTANICAL NAME	USES
1	Cassava flour	Farine de manioc	Manihot Utillissima	Tapioca Nkum-nkum Gari flour
2	Corn flour	Farine de mais	Zea mays	Corn foo foo Corn pap (bouilli de mais)
3	Colocasia flour	Farine de taro	Colocasia esculenta	Achu foo foo
4	Plantain flour	Farin de plantain	Musa sapientum var paradisiaca	Coating of fish
5	Millet flour	Farine de millet Farine de petit mil	Pennisetum Typhoideum	Bouilli de mil Goari (Fulbe)
6	Rice flour	Farine de riz	Oryza sativa	Rice foo foo Rice pap Couscous de riz Bouilli de riz
7	Sorghum flour	Farine de guinea Farine de gros mil	Sorghum vulgan	Guinea corn-foo foo
8	Sweet potato flour	Farine de patate		Baking bread
9	White Yam flour	Farine d'igname blanc		Yam foo foo

VEGETABLE CUTS

Cutting vegetables properly is very important because of these reasons

1. Uniformity in the sizes gives an attractive appearance.
2. Aesthetics: Food that is very attractive in appearance is highly appreciated.
3. Food cut evenly allows for even cooking.

THE BASIC TYPES OF CUTS

JULIENNE CUT: (MATCHSTICK CUT):

2mm x 2mm x 4cm.This is a type of stick-shape cut that is very thin. Carrots, zucchini, celery can be cut in julienne cut. Thin sticks with length and thickness of match sticks.

THE BRUNOISE DICE:

This is the smallest dice that can be obtained. 2mm x2mm x2mm. The julienne cut is bunched up in the hand. Then cut it into equally shaped dice. That is the brunoise, dice. It is also known as the fine dice. Carrots, onions, turnips used for sautéing or as a garnish for soups, meat, fish, or poultry dishes.

THE SMALL DICE: similar to the brunoise, but it is slightly larger 3mm x 3mm x 3mm

THE BATONNET:

Larger stick cut. Used when serving a larger portion of an item such as a vegetable side, to gain height in your dish or to provide imposing linear appeal to an otherwise linear absent dish. It is 6mm x 6mm x 6cm

THE MEDIUM DICE:

This is obtained from the batonnet. The batonnet is cut into cubes of 6mm x 6mm x 6mm

THE BATON (JARDINIÈRES):

It is the largest stick cut. It is used for crudités and for presentation purposes. It is the foundation for the more common large dice which is 12mm x 12mm x 6cm

THE LARGE DICE (MACEDOINE):

It is a cut used primarily for stews, long cooking dishes and for mirepoix in stocks. It is quick to cut, has an imposing nature and looks professional and measures 12mm x 12mm x 12mm melons and other fruits are cut using this cut.

THE PAYSANNE CUT:

It is a slimmer, flat, square can be squares, circles and/or diamonds. To do it you can create your desired stick-cut size, then slicing thinly to produce a thin square. Typically, it is used for larger cuts, but can be applied to smaller cuts and dices as well. It measures 12mm x 12mm x 3mm

THE CHIFFONADE (SHREDDING):

This cut is used when slicing very thin items such as herbs or leaf vegetables such as spinach, lettuce, cabbage, eru and herbs such as basil and mint. The items are stacked, rolled up, producing a cigar-shaped roll. Once rolled, start slicing to produce a nice chiffonade (ribbon) suitable for garnishing and other purposes. It is 1mm in thickness but vary in length.

SLICING:

Cutting food into thin, relatively broad slices used in many dishes from sandwiches through to meats. Sliced items may be processed further to produce cuts like chiffonade, tomatoes, peppers, lemons can be sliced.

MINCING:

Cutting the ingredients into thin strips, and then dicing the strips.

ROLL CUTTING: Used for long vegetables, like carrots, or zucchini. Cut on the diagonal, roll a quarter-turn, and cut down again at the same diagonal.

PARALLEL CUTTING: Used to cut broad, thin slices of meat or vegetables.

CRUSHING: Finely chopped e.g., ginger or garlic

MIREPOIX: Finely diced vegetables, often with the addition of bacon and herbs fried in butter and used as a basis for sauces. Carrots, celery, onions, are used for vegetable and meat stocks.

RUBANS: Thin, long, and broad slices, most often accomplished using a vegetable peeler and often used to add a decorative, elegant touch to any salad or dish.

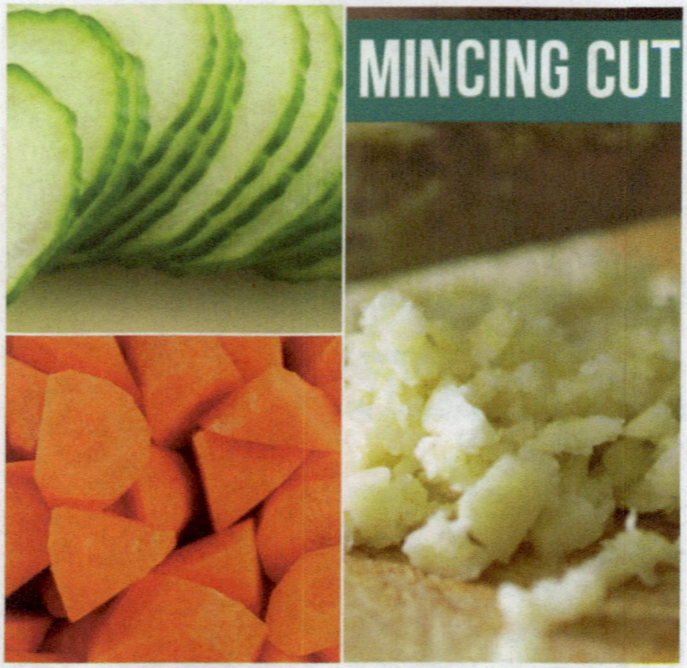

Slicing, mincing, roll cutting

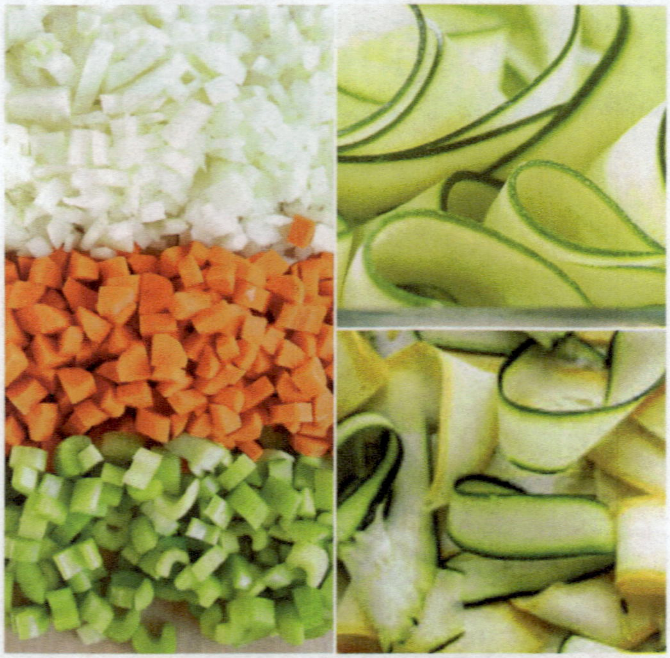

Mirepoix cutting, ruban (spiral) cut

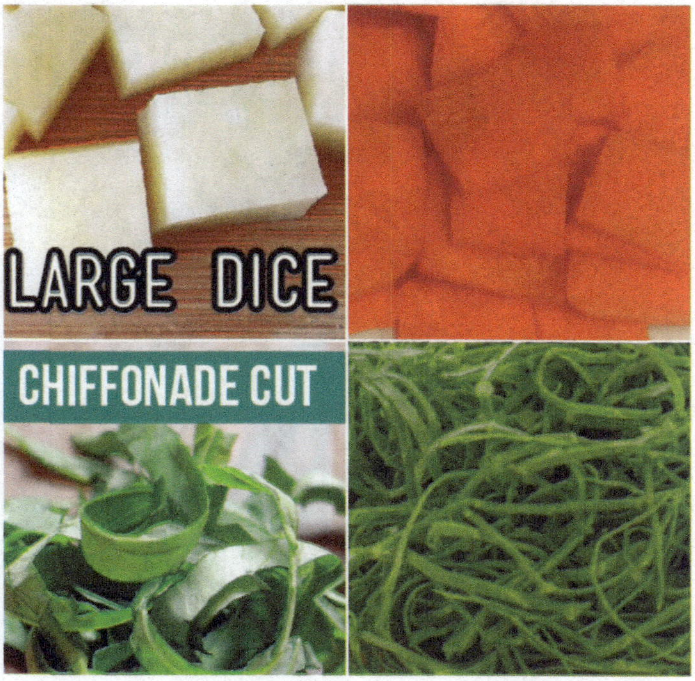

Large dice (macedoine), paysanne cut, chiffonnade (shredding)

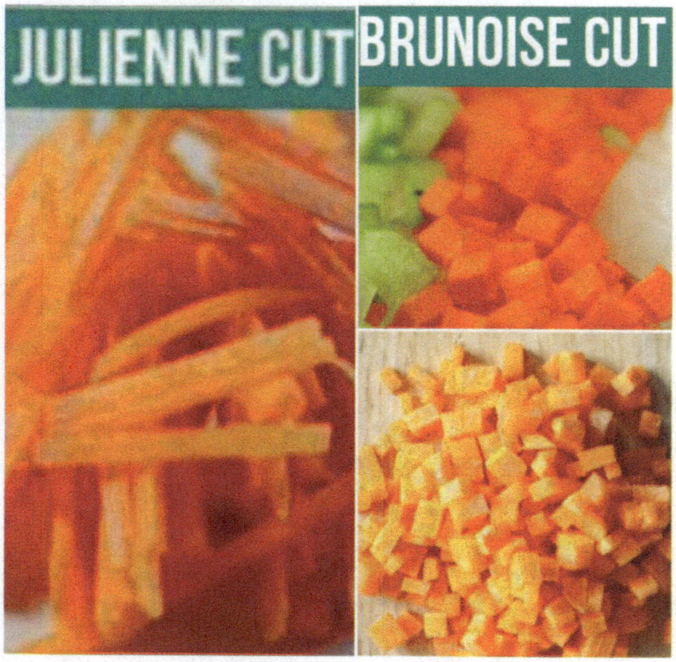

Julienne cut, brunoise cut, small dice.

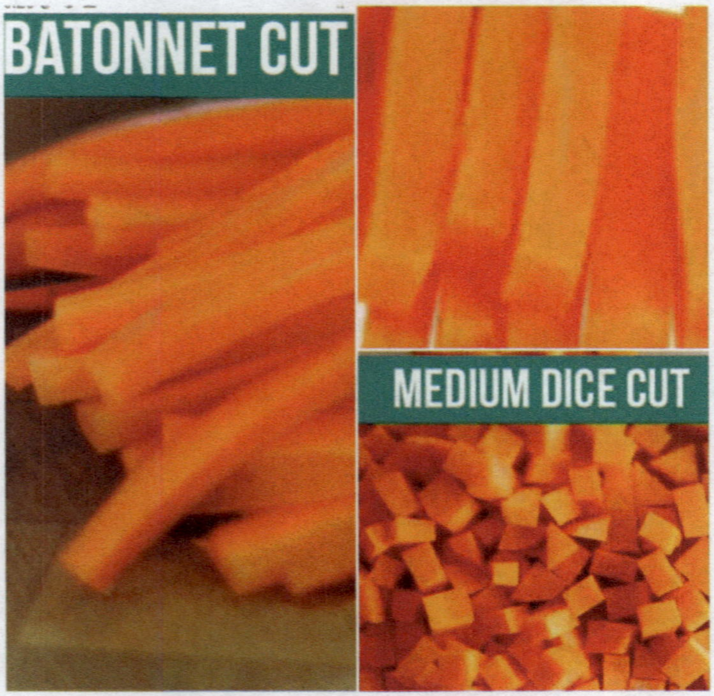

Batonnet cut, baton (jadiniere) cut, medium dice

THE HOSPITALITY INDUSTRY

Hospitality is the art of kindness in welcoming and looking after the basic needs of guests or strangers, mainly in relation to food, drinks, and accommodation.

The hospitality industry refers to the sector of the economy that includes businesses, companies or organizations that offer food and/or drinks and other services to people who are away from home. The increased demand by the international public for private function space outside their homes and businesses has made this industry the leader of the catering segment in growth and revenue. The services in this industry are lodging, accommodation services, restaurants, pubs, bars and clubs, hotels, contract catering, hospitable services, event planners, transportation, cruise line, gaming, entertainment and recreation, meeting and events, fast food outlets, care and nursing home, schools and prisons, armed forces, tourism services, and visitor information.

COMPONENTS OF THE TRAVEL AND TOURISM INDUSTRY

1. **Lodging operations:** Hotels, Motels, resorts camps, and parks.
2. **Food and Beverage operations:** Restaurants, Lodging properties, Bars/taverns, catering, snack bars, lunch counters, cruise ships, institutions, contract food companies.
3. **Transportation services:** Ships, airplanes, autos, buses, trains, bikes, limousines.
4. **Retail:** Gift shops.

CATERING

Catering is the art or business of providing food service at a remote site or site like a hotel, public house (pub), or other various locations. It is the provision of meals and snacks for groups of people. It involves the production, supply and service of food and drinks to guests at private parties or events. Catering involves a range of skills and duties, some creative; some hospitality-related catering is about satisfying all the senses of sight, hearing, touch, smell, and taste.

A caterer is any person/entity who supplies food and beverages and/or services to any off-premise public or private function. Food service or catering Industry is businesses, institutions, and companies responsible for any meal prepared outside the home.

Caterers work long hours, and even seven days a week during event seasons.

The tasks of a caterer are managing and completing budgets, designing menus for clients, producing food in large kitchens, traveling to deliver and serve food at different premises, organizing waiting staff, setting up and clearing at different venues, and building a client base and reputation. Caterers play an essential role in celebrating some of the most important occasions in people's lives. They work closely with event planners and private customers to design the perfect menus for a variety of events. Some caterers may specialize in a certain kind of cuisine, while others may work with a range of foods in a wide array of circumstances. Some caterers work in one-person operation, while others work for large companies. Every catering business is different. There will be different menu, different equipment, different system of drinks disperses and different methods of food preparation and service. There are two main types of catering.

TYPES OF CATERING

1. On-premises catering:

Is for any function – banquet, reception or event that is held on the physical premises of the establishment that is organizing/sponsoring the function. It takes place in a remote location, such as a client's home, a park, an art gallery, or even a parking lot, and the staff, food, and decor must be transported to that location. Some examples of on-premise catering include hospital catering, school, University/college catering.

2. Off- premises catering:

Involves producing food at a central kitchen, with delivery to and service provided at the client's location. Part or all of the production of food maybe executed or finished at the location of the event. There are three categories of off-premise catering:

Party food Caterers:

Supply only the food (cold food) for an event and leave the last-minute preparation, plus service and cleanup, to others.

Hot food Caterers:

Provide hot food from their commissaries in insulated containers. They sometimes provide serving personnel at an additional charge

Full-service Caterers:

They provide food, but frequently cook it to order on- site, provide service personnel, at the event, plus all food related equipment - china, glassware, flatware, cutleries, tables, and chairs, tents, and so forth. They can also arrange for other services like decor and music, as well. In short a full-service caterer can plan and execute an entire event, not just the food for it.

CATERING SEGMENTS

1. **Commercial segment:** For profit operations, Independent caterer, Restaurant caterer, Home-based caterer, and Hotel/motel and private clubs.
2. **Noncommercial segment:** Non-profit operation, Business/ industry accounts, College/University, social organizations, health care facilities, transportation food services, recreational food services (amusement and theme parks, conference and convention facilities, museums, libraries, stadium), and school catering.
3. **Military segment:** Armed forces and functions.

TYPES OF CATERING ESTABLISHMENTS

1. **Restaurant:** A restaurant is an establishment that serves the customers with prepared food and beverages to order, to be consumed on the premises.

2. **Transport Catering:** The provision of food and beverages to passengers, before, during, and after a journey on trains, aircrafts and ships, and in buses or private vehicles is termed as transport catering. These services may also be utilized by the general public, who are in the vicinity of the transport catering unit. **3. Outdoor catering:**

3. The provision of food and drink away from home base and supplies. Outdoor catering includes catering functions such marriages, parties, and conventions. The venue is left to the people's choice. The type of food and set-up depends entirely on the price agreed upon.

4. **Retail Store Catering:** Some retail stores, apart from carrying on their primary activity of retailing their own wares, provide catering as an additional facility.

5. **Club Catering:** Refers to the provision of food and beverages to a restricted clientele e.g., clubs with people of similar interests such as golf clubs, cricket club, veteran club etc.

6. **Welfare Catering:** The provision of food and beverages to people, who fulfil a social obligation, determined by a recognized authority e.g., catering for hospitals, schools, colleges, the armed forces, and prisons.

7. **Industrial Catering:** The provision of food and beverages to people at work, in industries and factories at highly subsidized rates.

8. **Leisure-linked Catering:** The provision of food and beverages to people engaged in 'rest and recreation' activities. This includes the sale of food and beverages through different stalls and kiosks at exhibitions, theme parks, galleries, and theatres. Catering can also be classified as Social cratering and corporate or business catering.

SOCIAL CATERING: Events like weddings, bar mitzvahs, high school reunions, birthday parties, and charity events.

BUSINESS CATERING: Association conventions and meetings, civic meetings, corporate sales of stockholder meetings, recognition banquets, product launches, educational training sessions, seller-buyer meets, service awards banquets, and entertaining in hospitality suites.

SCOPE OF THE CATERING SECTOR

Banqueting, Clubs, Contract catering, Hotel and Guest houses, Full-service restaurants, Catering Halls, Independent caterers, Boxed lunch catering, Event catering, Mobile catering, Charcuteries and Delicatessens, takeaway and fast-food restaurants, food on the move (trains, coaches, boats, airplanes), Fish and Chips restaurants, and Public Houses.

SKILLS OF A CATERER

1. **CULINARY ABILITY AND CREATIVITY:** A caterer should be able to produce large quantity of food and collaborate with customers to put together the right menu for the right events. Be a flexible cook.

2. **SOCIAL SKILLS:** Be able to attract customers and sell your product. Be prepared to meet the demands of a client. Listen to them and be able to deliver the food and services they want on time and in good condition.

3. **BUSINESS SKILLS:** Have a good sense of cost. Be able to work with customers within their budgets. Also figure out your own budgets and pricing, i.e., be able to manage your own accounts, deal with staff issues, maintaining a contact list and working in a team to deliver a professional and consistent service. Being prepared and well-ordered will ensure that things run effectively, and a good service is delivered.

THINGS THAT DISTINGUISH A CATERING OPERATION FROM A RESTAURANT.

1. Catering is usually done by prearranged contract.

2. Food and drink is provided at a certain cost to a specific number of people

3. The menu at a catered event is usually more limited than a restaurant menu and is chosen in advance by a client.

4. The way the food is cooked is different from that of the restaurant in that, catering chefs prepare their food so that it needs brief final cooking, reheating, or assembly prior to service.

CATERING MENU PRICES

COSTS AND PROFIT

PROFIT: is the portion of revenue that remains after all operating costs are paid.

COSTS: are all expenses required to conduct business, including rent or mortgage, taxes, licensing fee, and contracts such as laundry, pest control, equipment service and thrash removal, plus food, labor, supplies, telephone, heat, electricity, water, advertising, and printing, to name a few. Cost is broken into three major categories:

1. **Food- and- beverage cost**: The cost of all food-related purchases required to produce completed menu items.
2. **Labor Costs:** The cost associated with labor, including benefits, taxes, wages, meals, and uniforms.
3. **Overhead costs:** The costs of operating the business. To these three costs can be added profit:
4. **Profit:** funds remaining after all costs have been paid from revenue. In the average food service operation, these four factors generally are located in the diagram shown.

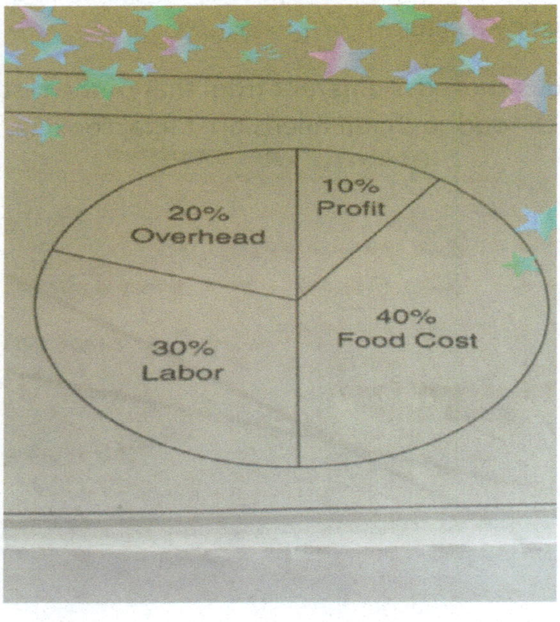

RESTAURANTS

A restaurant is a retail establishment that serves prepared food to customers. Service is or eating is on premises, though the term has been used to include take-out establishments and food delivery services. A successful restaurant is one which the guests are anxious to visit again. Good waiters are necessary for the success and development of the restaurant. The waiter is in direct contact with guests and therefore much of restaurant's success depends on the skills, interest, and personal qualities of the waiter.

The waiter is also known as a steward or Commis-de-rang. The duties of the waiter include the preparing tables (table setting) for a meal, taking customers' orders, serving drinks and food, and cleaning up before, during and after servings in a restaurant.

The quality of any serving staff in any establishment reflects the quality of the establishment itself. The important qualities of a waiter are personal hygiene and appearance, good conduct, good memory, observation, concentration and skill, salesmanship, ability to assume responsibility, maximize revenue, punctuality, local knowledge, personality, attitude to customers, honesty, etc.

CLASSIFICATION OF RESTAURANTS

They are classified by whether they provide places to sit, whether they are served by wait-staff and quality of the service, the formal atmosphere, and the price range. Restaurants are generally classified into three groups:

1. **QUICK SERVICE:** Also known as fast food restaurants and offer limited menus that are prepared quickly. They may be self-service outlets and drive- thru windows and take-out.
2. **MID SCALE:** They offer full meals at a medium price that customers perceive as 'good value'. They can be of full service, buffets, or limited service with customers ordering at the counter and having their food brought to them or self-service.
3. **UPSCALE:** Offer high quality cuisine at a high-end price. They offer full service and have a high quality of ambiance.

TYPES OF RESTAURANTS

1. *CAFETERIAS*:

A cafeteria is a restaurant serving mostly cooked ready to eat food, arranged behind a food serving counter. There is little or no table service. Typically, a patron takes a tray and pushes it along a track in front of the counter. Depending on the establishment, servings may be ordered from attendants, selected as ready-made portions already on plates, or self-service of food of their own choice. In some establishments, a few items such as steaks maybe ordered specially prepared rare, medium, and well done from the attendants. The patron waits for those items to be prepared or is given a number and they will be brought to the table. Beverages may be filled from self-service dispensers or ordered from the attendants. At the end of the line a cashier rings up the purchases. At some self-service cafeterias, purchases are priced by weight, rather than by individual item. The trays filled with selected items of food are taken to a table to eat. Institutional cafeterias may have common tables, but upscale cafeterias have traditional cutlery and crockery, and some have servers to carry the trays from the line to the patrons' tables, and/or bus the empty trays and used dishes. Cafeterias have a wider variety of prepared foods. For example, it may have a variety of roast (beef, ham, turkey) ready for carving by the server, as well as other cooked entrees, rather than simply an offering of hamburgers or fried chicken.

2. *FAST-FOOD RESTAURANTS*:

They emphasize speed of service and low cost over all other considerations. A feature of newer fast-food restaurants is the lack of cutlery or crockery; the customer is expected to eat the food directly from the disposable container it was served in using their fingers.

Types of fast-food restaurants:

a. One collects food from a counter and pays, then sits down and starts eating (as a self-service restaurant or cafeterias).

b. One collects ready portions.

c. One serves oneself from containers

d. One is served at the counter.

e. A special procedure is that one first pays at the cash desk, collects a coupon, and then goes to the food counter, where one gets the food in exchange for the coupon.

f. One orders at the counter, after preparation the food is brought to one's table, paying may be on ordering or after eating.

g. A drive-through is a type of fast-food restaurant without seating; diners receive their food and most fast-food restaurants offer take-out, ready-to-eat hot food in disposable packaging for the customer to eat off-site.

3. *CASUAL RESTAURANTS*:

Is a restaurant that serves moderately priced food in a casual atmosphere. Except for buffet style restaurants, casual dining restaurants typically provide table service. Casual dining comprises a market segment between fast food establishments and fine dining restaurants.

4. *FAST CASUAL-DINING RESTAURANTS*:

A fast casual-dining restaurant is similar to a fast- food restaurant in that it does not offer full- service but promises a somewhat higher quality of food and atmosphere. Average prices charged are higher than fast- food prices and non- disposable plates and cutlery are usually offered. It fills the space between fast food and casual dining. Counter service accompanied by handmade food, often visible via an open kitchen. Alcohol may be served. Dishes like steak, which require experience on the part of one cook to get it right, may be offered. The menu is usually limited to an extended over-counter display, and options in the way the food is prepared are emphasized. Many fast casual-dining restaurants are marketed as health-conscious: healthy items may have a larger number of items than normal portion of the menu and high-quality ingredients such as free-range chicken and freshly made salsas may be advertised. Overall, the quality of the food is presented as a much higher class than conventional factory-made fast food. An ethnic theme may or may not be present in the menu.

5. *OTHER RESTAURANTS*:

Most of these establishments can be considered as subtypes of fast casual-dining restaurants or casual-dining restaurant:

a. **Café:** Cafes and coffee shops are informal restaurants offering a range of hot meals and made- to-order sandwiches. Cafes offer table service. Many cafes are open for breakfast and serve full hot breakfasts. In some areas, cafes offer outdoor seating.

b. **Coffeehouse:** Are casual restaurants without table service emphasizing coffee and other beverages; typically, a limited selection of cold foods such as pastries and perhaps sandwiches are offered as well. Their distinguishing feature is that they allow patrons to relax and socialize on their premises for long periods of time without pressure to leave promptly after eating.

c. **Pub:** (short for public house): Is a bar that serves food fare. Traditionally, pubs were primarily drinking establishments with food in a decidedly secondary position, whereas the modern pub business relies on food as well, to the point where gastropubs are known for their high-quality pub food. A typical pub has a large selection of beers and ales on tap.

d. **Bistros and Brasseries:** A brasserie is a café doubling as a restaurant and serving single dishes and other meals in a relaxing setting. A bistro is a familiar name for a café serving moderately priced simple meals in an unpretentious setting. Especially in Paris, bistros have become increasingly popular with tourists. When used in English, the term bistro usually indicates either a fast casual-dining restaurant with a European-influenced menu or a café with a larger menu of food.

e. **Family Style:** Family style restaurant" are restaurants those that have a fixed menu and fixed price, usually with diners seated at a communal table such as on bench seats. There is no menu to choose from; rather food is brought out in courses, usually with communal serving dishes, like at a family meal.

f. **BYO Restaurants:** These are restaurants and bistros which do not have a liquor license.

g. **Delicatessens Restaurants:** Restaurants offering food for immediate consumption. The main product line is normally luncheon meats and cheeses. They may offer sandwiches, soups, and salad as well. Most foods are precooked prior to delivery. Preparation of food products is generally simple and only involves one or two steps.

h. **Ethnic Restaurants:** They range from quick service to upscale. Their menus usually include ethnic dishes and/or authentic foods. Specialize in a particular multicultural cuisine not specifically accommodated by any other listed categories. Example: Cameron cuisine, Chinese cuisine, Indian cuisine, American cuisine etc.

6. *DESTINATION RESTAURANTS*:

A destination restaurant is one that has a strong enough appeal to draw customers from beyond its community. Example: Michelin Guide 3-star restaurant in Europe, which according to the restaurant guides is "worthy of a journey"

TABLE SETTING

Table setting refers to the way to set a table with tableware- such as eating utensils and dishware for serving and eating. Table setting is an art. The arrangement for a single diner is called a place setting. A **cover** is a place setting for one person. It is the area or space for all utensils (including salt, pepper cruets, and ash trays), for each guest. It should be approximately 60cm by 38cm preferably. The arrangement varies across various cultures. The rules for laying a table are not rigid. They are followed to facilitate dining and making the tables neat.

BASIC RULES FOR LAYING THE TABLES

1. **Table linens:** Table linen has to be laid properly. A white cloth is preferred but not mandatory. The only rule is to make sure that linen patterns don't clash.

2. **Chargers:** Chargers are decorative elements that are placed underneath plates to add color or texture to the plate. Chargers or dinner plates should be placed on the table first. Each plate should be set in the center of the place setting and each place setting on the table should be set equidistant. The rest of the components used to set a formal table will be set with the dinner plate in mind. If a charger is used, soup and melon bowls will be placed on top. The charger will generally be removed just before the main course.

3. **Napkins:** Linen napkins should be folded elegantly and placed in the center of the dinner plate or in between the cutlery. Normally during a dinner session, napkins are arranged in empty water tumblers.

4. **Silverware:** Silverware is to be placed in order of use. In other words, the diner will start at the end and work his way in. The first course will use silver ware farthest from the dinner plate, while the last course will utilize the silverware closest. Place all silverware 3cm from the table's edge.

5. **Knives:** Set knives on the table to the right of the dinner plate. Technically, one should only use a knife if one is cutting meat; however up to three knives can be placed on the table in order of use, from outside towards the inner setting, with blades facing towards the plates.

6. **Forks:** Forks are to be set to the left of the dinner plate in order of use. In most cases there are three; one each for seafood, the main course, and the salad. When dining formally, salads are generally served at the end of the meal.

7. **Spoons:** Spoons are set to the right of the knives in order of use. If there is a melon course, this spoon will be set closest to the plate with soup spoon on the end. If there is a dessert spoon, this will be set above the plate. Coffee spoons are set on the saucer when it's time for dessert.

8. **Glasses:** Glasses are set above the plate to the right in order of use. From the left to the right, Water glass, red wine glass, white wine glass, champagne flute (if ordered).

9. **Dessert:** Dessert plates and coffee/teacups will be set out after dinner. If a fork is to be used with dessert, this will be placed on the dessert plate. A dessert spoon should have already been set above the dinner plate. Coffee spoons should be placed on the saucer. Coffee/tea mugs aren't used for formal dinner.

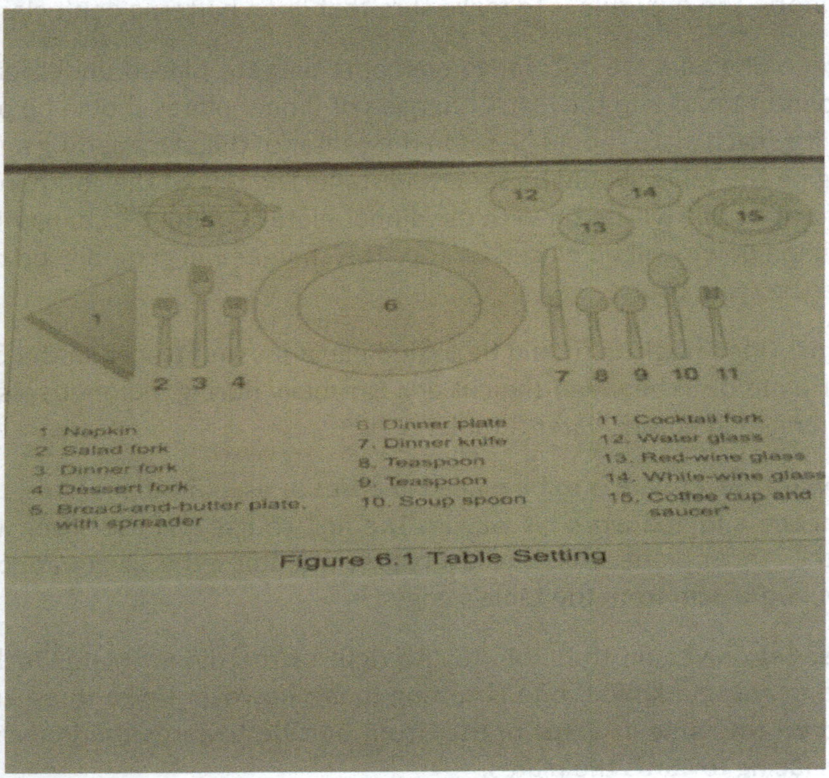

Figure 6.1 Table Setting

EQUIPMENT FOR SETTING A TABLE

1. ***TABLECLOTH*: Attractive colors, but white is ever popular. Most commonly made of cotton or linen, rayon or rayon blend are attractive and launder well and can be plastic coated. Great deals of designs go well with plain dishes. Plain dishes go with figured or plain cloth. Tablecloths should not hang more than 30cm over the edge of the table.**

2. ***MOLTON* (baize base cloth):** The molton is the same size of the table. The baize base cloth protects the diner's wrists and elbows from the table's sharp edges, keeps the tablecloth firmly in place, protects the surface of the table and prevents the rattling of crockery and cutlery and to absorb moisture in case liquid spills on the table.

3. ***NAPERONES OR SLIP CLOTH*:** The naperone is placed diagonally to the tablecloth to protect it from spillage and gives it a longer life. The four edges of the naperone hang down equally on each side. Slip cloths measure 1metre square approximately.

4. ***NAPKINS OR SERVIETTES*:** They can be paper or cloth. The color of napkins should blend with the tablecloth and with other color schemes. The ideal size for a napkin is between 46 to 50 sq cm.

5. ***PLACE MATS*:** They should be colorful, easy to care for, made of cotton, linen, plastic, cork, or bamboo. For hot food, insulator mats will be used.

6. ***DISHES*:** China refers to all types of dishes. China is the most fragile looking, yet the strongest of the materials used to make dishes. It is also referred to as porcelain. It is the choicest of dish materials because it does not crack, break nor chip readily as pottery or earthen ware. It is expensive but lasts for a long time.
    - **Earthen ware:** It is made of less refined material. It cracks and chips more easily than china. It is used for everyday dishes.
    - **Pottery:** It is a thick, heavy earthen ware made of crude clay. It often has a rough texture and tends to chip and breaks easily. It is a popular type of everyday dinner ware.
    - **Plastic:** It is of many varieties and qualities. Some are thin and easily heat- warped or cracked, and stain, others are very strong, maybe plain or patterned. In many instances they look like china.

7. ***SILVER WARE*:**A term applied to eating utensils. Eating utensils called flatware (serving spoons & serving forks) maybe made of silver or silver plated but may also be made of stainless steel or even plastic.

- **Sterling silver:** Is the most expensive. Sterling means that it is made of 92.5% silver with the rest and alloy to give hardness.
- **Vermeil:** Flat ware made of silver gilded with gold.
- **Silver plate:** Flat ware made of some metal usually covered with a coat of silver.
- **Triple plate:** It has three layers of silver coating.
- **Stainless steel flat ware**: Most acceptable everyday utensil material. It does not tarnish or stain and does not require polishing.
- **Plastics:** Used mainly for picnics

8. ***GLASS WARE***: It is the term applied to table items (glasses and drink ware)
    - **Crystal:** This is the most delicate and beautiful of glass ware. It has a superior, colorless, clear brilliancy. Crystal maybe of any thickness. Glass ware comes in a variety of colors as well as clear. Use colors which blend well with the dishes, cloth, or mats. Heavy glass ware goes a little better with pottery or earthen ware dishes than a fragile glass. Thin crystal is more elegant with delicate china.
    - **Glass ware** (glass and drink ware for red wine, white wine, and water)
    - **Table ware** (Dishes, glass ware, cutlery, flat ware)
    - **Flat ware** (spoons and forks)
    - **Cutlery** (knives and other cutting instruments)
    - **Hollow ware** (sugar bowls, creamers, coffee pots, tea pots and soup tureens)
    - **Silver wear** (serving spoons and forks)
    - **Reserves** (tablecloth naperones napkins serving cloths, molton)
    - **China** (crockery i.e., casserole, and oven proof ware, dishes, cocotte dishes), plates for cold dishes, big, small and bread plates, plate for hot dishes, and cups which are kept in warmers)

9. ***SERVING PIECES***: Place serving spoons beside the serving dishes. The butter knife and sugar spoon should be beside the butter dish and sugar bowl.

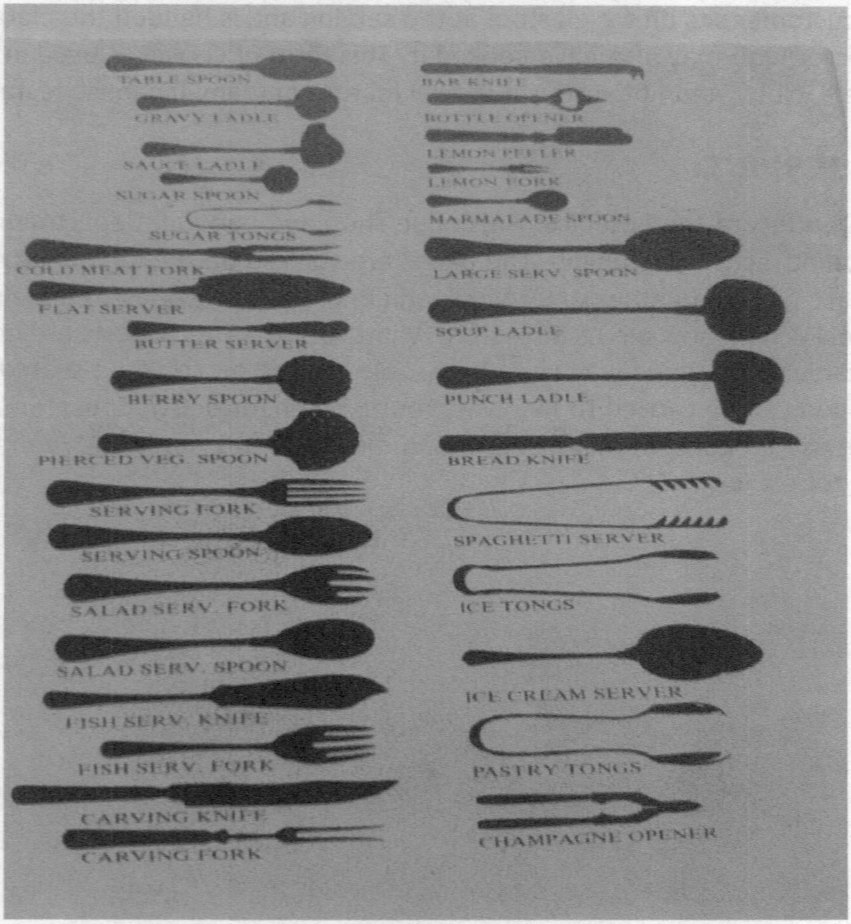
TABLE SPOON
GRAVY LADLE
SAUCE LADLE
SUGAR SPOON
SUGAR TONGS
COLD MEAT FORK
FLAT SERVER
BUTTER SERVER
BERRY SPOON
PIERCED VEG. SPOON
SERVING FORK
SERVING SPOON
SALAD SERV. FORK
SALAD SERV. SPOON
FISH SERV. KNIFE
FISH SERV. FORK
CARVING KNIFE
CARVING FORK
BAR KNIFE
BOTTLE OPENER
LEMON PEELER
LEMON FORK
MARMALADE SPOON
LARGE SERV. SPOON
SOUP LADLE
PUNCH LADLE
BREAD KNIFE
SPAGHETTI SERVER
ICE TONGS
ICE CREAM SERVER
PASTRY TONGS
CHAMPAGNE OPENER

SELF SERVICE STYLES

CAFETERIA SERVICE AND COUNTER SERVICE:

It is the most widely used method. All fast-food outlets and commercial cafeterias are self service outlets: Cafeteria service and counter service. A special type of counter service is where the customer sits on a high stool at the serving and is handed the plate of food by the food server who may also have cooked it. This form of service is used in snack bars, supermarkets, clubs, and hotels. It is a special feature of many Japanese restaurants.

BUFFET SERVICE:

It is used in outlets of the hotel like the coffee shop and banquet department. A table is set with food attractively arranged. The plates are stacked on the table. The napkins and silver ware are placed together, and the beverage, the cups and glasses are also arranged on the table. Each person serves himself to whatever he wants. Guests are not seated at the buffet table. It is a good way to serve people more than could be seated at a dining table. The food can be carried to the living room, porch, or out-of-doors. Small tables or trays maybe used. People at a large reception may wish to stand if the food to be eaten does not require a fork.

TABLE SERVICE STYLES

FAMILY SERVICE OR ENGLISH SERVICE:

It originated in the home and is used mainly in family restaurants or coffee shops. All the food is put in dishes and bowls in the kitchen by the food production staff and placed in the center of the dining table by the service staff. The guests serve themselves from dishes and bowls of food placed in the center of the table by the service staff.

PLATE SERVICE OR AMERICAN SERVICE:

It is portioning the food on a dinner plate in the kitchen. It is less formal, fastest of all table service, most widely used table service style, used in most inexpensive and average priced restaurants, such as family restaurants, pub restaurants and coffee shops. Plating of food is done in gastronomique restaurants for certain dishes.

SILVER SERVICE OR RUSSIAN SERVICE OR FORMAL STYLE SERVICE:

Food is cooked and proportioned in the kitchen and presented to the guests on silver platter by the service staff. The food is served from the platter onto the guest's plates, which is already placed infront of the guest. This service originated in Russia and was used in the household of the rich aristocrats. To make the food look attractive as possible it was served from silver platters which were the best serving pieces. Russian service, sometimes called platter service is well suited for banquet service, because the food stays hotter and longer when served from silver platter. Used in "high style" entertainment or formal banquets. A waitress is needed for every four to six people. The food is served entirely from the kitchen. Two types of formal service:

- **PLATTER SERVICE:** The food is arranged attractively on platters or in serving dishes. The waitress holds the serving dish at the person's left so that each individual may serve himself or the waitress may serve the guests.
- **PLATE SERVICE:** All food is placed on the plates in the kitchen and the waitress serves a plate individually to each person, course by course.

GUERIDON SERVICE OR FRENCH SERVICE:

The highest level is the gueridon service or French service. This is the style traditionally used in gastronomique restaurants. The word gueridon means a side table or mobile table such as a trolley which is brought close to the guest's dinner table. Any carving or finishing of the food is done in front of the guest. Only skilled or well-trained are allowed to do this form of service as a good knowledge of food preparation is required in addition to the service style.

***BUTLER SERVICE*:**

This is a very personal type of room service provided by highly trained waiters. It is only offered in more exclusive hotels and resorts. A butler is on standby and assigned to only a specific number of rooms. Besides the service of food and beverages, they will assist the guest with small tasks, such as packing and unpacking their suitcase or pressing clothes.

FOOD PRESENTATION

Food presentation is the art of modifying, processing, arranging and decorating food to enhance its aesthetic appeal.

Visual presentation of foods at many different stages of food preparation can depend on:

1. The manner of tying or sewing meats
2. The type of cut use in chopping and slicing meats or vegetables.
3. The kind of mold used in a poured dish
4. Edible or inedible garnishes
5. Decorated foods itself as in elaborately iced cakes topped with ornamental sculptural consumables, drizzled with sauces, sprinkled with seeds, powder or other toppings.

FOOD PLATING

The arrangement and overall styling of food upon bringing it to the plate is called food plating. The goal of plating food is to create a dining-experience that tempts all of the senses.

In plating food, the following points are necessary.

1. Avoid monochromatic color scheme.
2. Bring out vegetables brightest colors by steaming vegetables, roast, or sauté with a little oil or butter.
3. Sear meat and let it rest.
4. Experiment with interesting shapes
5. Limit portion sizes. Only fill 2/3 of each plate with food. The rest of the plate should be left empty.
6. The negative space will provide contrast with a starch.

THE BASIC ELEMENTS OF FOOD PLATING

PICK THE PLATE:

The size, shape and color of a plate will have a direct impact on the overall appearance of your dish. White is a popular color because it creates a high contrast when paired with other colors, which means that your food will be the focus rather than the afterthought.

CREATE A FRAMEWORK:

Start with drawings and sketches to visualize the plate.

FIND A FOCAL POINT:

Select a focal point when plating your dish and is usually the protein. Use space to simplify the presentation. Other aspects of the dish such as accompanying vegetable, sauce, and garnishes, and even the plate itself will play supporting roles to the main attraction.

BALANCE THE DISH:

Play with colors, shapes, and textures to ensure that the diners are not overwhelmed. Draw attention to the positives of the meal by juxtaposing bright accent colors with more neutral tones. The texture of food creates an immediate attraction to the eye. Keep a plate visually stimulating by pairing such contrasting textures with one another, which also creates an intriguing textural contrast in each bite. The presentation should never empower flavor and function.

AIM HIGH: Height in plating helps to draw the eyes up and towards the focal point of a dish.

GET THE RIGHT PORTION SIZE:

Ensure that there is the right amount of ingredients and that the plate compliments the dish, not too big or too small a plate. Strike the right portion of protein, carbohydrates, and vegetables to create a nutritionally balanced meal.

ODDS RULE: Groupings of three, five or seven are naturally more appealing to the eye in that the lack of balance creates visual interest.

GARNISH WITH A PURPOSE:

All garnishes on a plate should both have a purpose and edible. Avoid using parsley flowers, lemon twists, cinnamon sticks, or raw herbs. Garnishes serve as an accent to perk up or highlight the color of the main dish. It is meant to enhance and match the flavors of the dish, not overpower it. Refrain from heaping garnishes on one corner of the plate. Do not garnish with a food that is not included in the recipe.

PROVIDE A FLASH OF COLOUR AND SHAPE:

By arranging the garnishes around a main dish. Garnishes should be applied quickly to ensure that the food arrives the table warm.

CLEANLINESS COUNTS:

Keep your plate clean by wiping away crumbs or dribble sauce. Such outliers will distract from the focal point and create a less polished look to your plate. Food should be plated on warmed plates.

THE PLATING PROCESS

CREATE A CLOCK:

The classical plating technique uses the three basic food items of starch, vegetables, and meat in a specific arrangement. A simple guide to a classical plating is to think of the plate as the face of a clock.

MAIN (PROTEIN): Between 3 to 9 o'clock

STARCH: Between 9 to 11 o'clock

VEGETABLES: Between 11 to 3 o'clock.

1. The plating using a clock face can also place protein at 6 o'clock, starch at 11:00 and vegetables at 2 o'clock.
2. The most attractive food is placed at the front of the plate.
3. Start plating food in the center of the plate and work outward from there, so that the food is centered in the middle of the plate. ½ of the food on the plate should comprise vegetables, ¼ should be starch and ¼ should comprise meat or other protein.
4. One-dish meals: The starch is usually plated in the center, topped with protein and vegetables placed around the sides. Balance the color and texture of these dishes.
5. Molded ingredients: Cleverly cut or sculptured ingredients can enhance the visual appeal of dishes. Slice filet of meat at a bias to show doneness and quality. Sculptured food provides height and structure and keeps the plate neat and clean.
6. Sauces: Sauces create accents in the form of dots on the side of the plate or as a character on one side of the plate. When applying a sauce, lightly pour or drizzle it on the plate either over the dish or underneath.

PLATING TYPES

1. **THE CLASSIC ARRANGEMENT**: Main item in front of the plate with vegetables or starches in the back.
2. **STACKED ARRANGEMENT** of various items or a main item leaning or "shingled" upon a vegetable bed or side item.

COMPONENTS OF GREAT FOOD STYLING

FOOD PRESENTATION

THE SUPPORT: Plain white plates

THE FOCAL POINT: The thing that will attract the eye, most voluminous, piece of meat or fish.

COLOURS: Green brings coolness and calms down, Red stands for passion and excitement Blue is a natural appetite suppressant and makes food unappetizing.

FLAVOURS

TEXTURES: firm and soft, silky, and rigid contrasts.

DECORATION: Must be edible and can be herbs, spices, or ingredients.

GARNISH: Increases the texture and flavor of the dish.

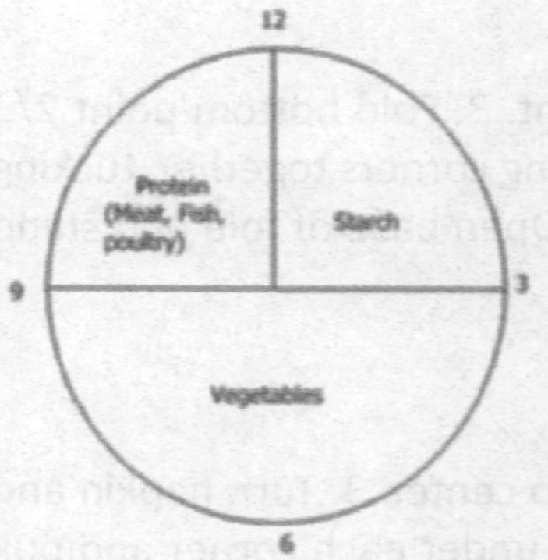

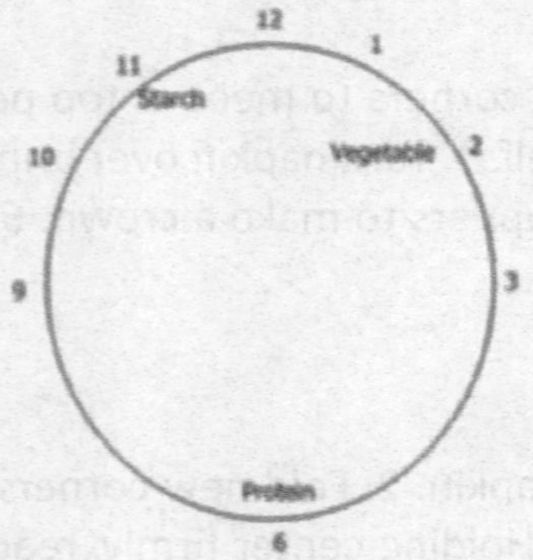

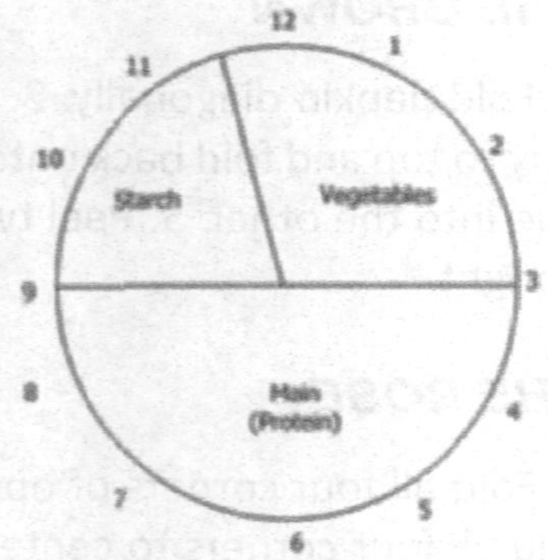

CLASSICAL PLATING CLOCK **CLASSICAL PLATING CLOCK 2** **FOOD SERVING CLOCK**

TABLE NAPKIN FOLDING
METHODS OF FOLDING NAPKINS

BISHOP'S MITRE

1. Fold napkin bringing top to bottom. 2. Fold corners to center line. 3. Turn napkin over and rotate ¼ turn. 4. Fold bottom edge up to top edge and flip point out from under top fold. 5. Turn left end into pleat at left forming a point on left side. 6. Turn napkin over and turn right end into pleat forming a point on right side. 7. Open base and stand upright.

ROSEBUD

1. Fold napkin in half diagonally. 2. Fold corners to meet at top point. 3. Turn napkin over and fold bottom 2/3 way up. 4. Turn napkin around and bring the corners together; tucking one into the other. 5. Turn napkin around and stand on the base.

PYRAMID

1. Fold napkin in half diagonally. 2. Fold corners to meet top point. 3. Turn napkin over and fold in half. 4. Pick up at center and stand on base of triangle.

THE CROWN

1. Fold napkin diagonally. 2. Fold corners to meet at top point. 3. Fold bottom point 2/3 way to top and fold back onto itself. 4. Turn napkin over bringing corners together, tucking one into the other. 5. Peel two toppers to make a crown. 6. Open base of fold and stand upright.

THE ROSE

1. Fold all four corners of open napkin. 2. Fold new corners to center. 3. Turn napkin and fold all four corners to center. 4. Holding center firmly, reach under each corner and pull up flaps to form petals. 5. Reach between petals and pull flaps from under.

LADY WINDERMERE'S FAN

1. Fold napkin in half. 2. Make 1.5cm accordion pleats, starting at bottom. 3. Fold in half with pleating on the outside. 4. Fold upper right corner diagonally down to folded base of pleats and turn under edge. 5. Place on table and release pleats to form fan.

THE CLOWN'S HAT

1. Fold napkin in half bringing bottom to top. 2. Holding center of bottom with finger, take lower right corner and loosely roll around center, matching corners, until cone is formed. 3. Turn napkin upside down, then turn them all around. 4. Turn and stand on base.

ARUM LILY

1. Fold napkin bringing bottom up to top. 2. Fold corners to top. 3. Fold bottom point up to 1 inch below top. 4. Fold point back unto itself. 5. Fold down each of points at top and tuck under edge of folded up bottom. Fold down one layer of top point and tuck under base fold. 6. Turn napkin over and tuck left and right sides into each. 7. Open base and stand.

CARDINAL'S HAT

1. Fold napkin in half diagonally. 2. Fold corners to meet at top point. 3. Turn napkin over with points to the top, fold lower corner 2/3 way up. 4. Fold back onto itself. 5. Bring corners together tucking one into the other. 6. Open base of fold and stand upright.

BIRD OF PARADISE

1. Fold napkin in half, and then half again diagonally. 2. Then fold in half diagonally with points on top and facing up. 3. Fold left and right sides down along center line, turning their extended points under. 4. Fold points of bottom corners underneath and fold in half on long end. 5. Pull up points and arrange fabric on a surface.

FLEUR DE LYS GOBLET FOLD

1. Lay the napkin face down Infront of you. 2. Fold the napkin in half diagonally.
3. Orient the napkin so that the open-end points towards you. 4. Fold the bottom points up so that the tip overlays the far edge by about 1.5cm. 5. Accordion fold the entire napkin from left to right. 6. Firmly grasp the base and insert it into a glass or a napkin ring.

LILY GOBLET

1. Lay the napkin face down in front of you. 2. Fold the napkin in front of you. 3. Fold the napkin into quarters. 4. Accordion fold the entire napkin from corner to corner. 5. Fold the napkin into half. 6. Tuck the napkin into a glass of your choice. 7. Using your finger, gently pull apart the loose corners sticking up, so that they are evenly distributed.

THE CANDLE FAN FOLD

1. Lay the napkin face down Infront of you. 2. Fold both sides in so that they meet at the center. Press the folds down well. 3. Take each of the four corners (one sitting at the center) of the far and near sides and fold them diagonally pivoting at the center of the napkin. 4. Starting at the end, tightly roll the napkin halfway along its length. The tighter, the better. 5. Accordion fold the other side of the napkin and gather ii together. 6. Fold the napkin in half and with the roll in the middle. 7. Place it into your goblet.

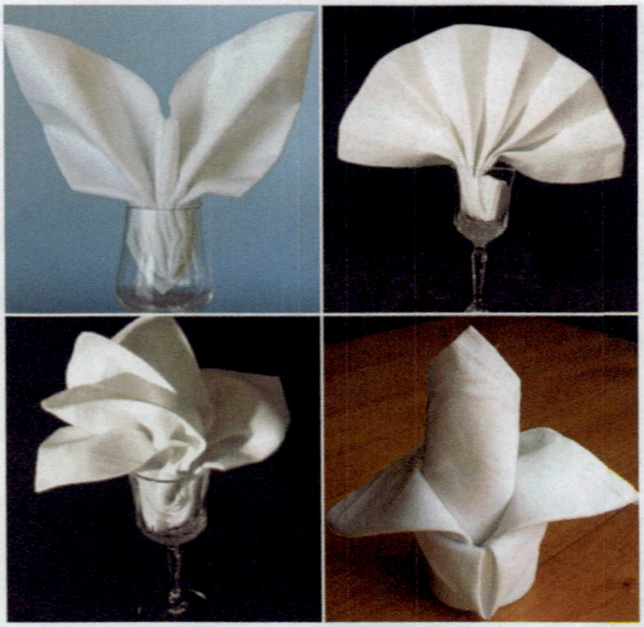

Lily fold, the lady Windermer fan fold, the Goblet lily fold, the crown fold.

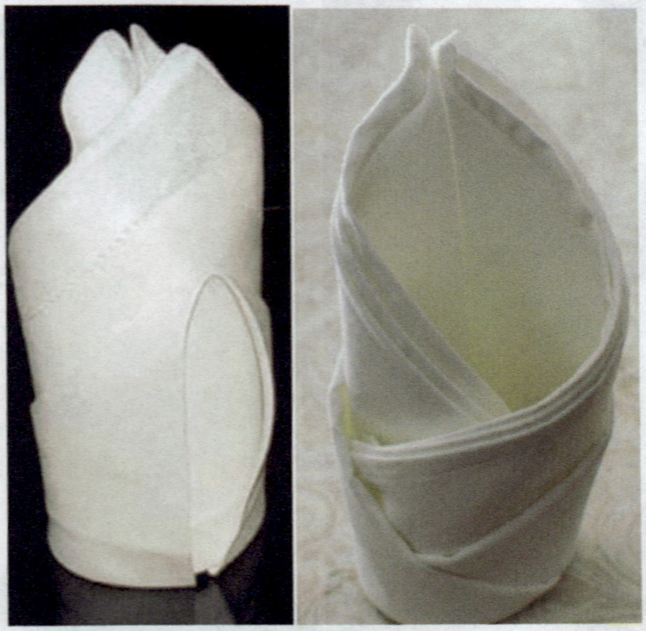

The Rose bud fold

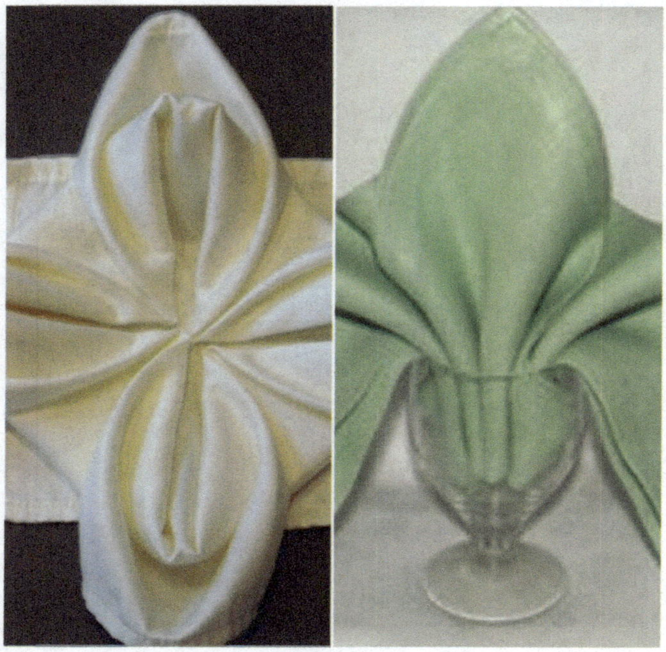

Rose flower fold, fleur de lys napkin fold.

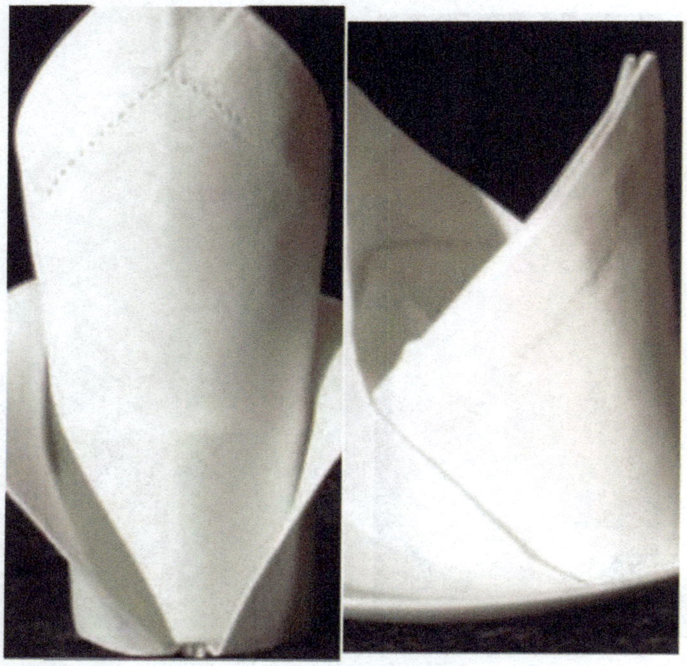

Cardinal's hat fold, Bishop's mitre fold

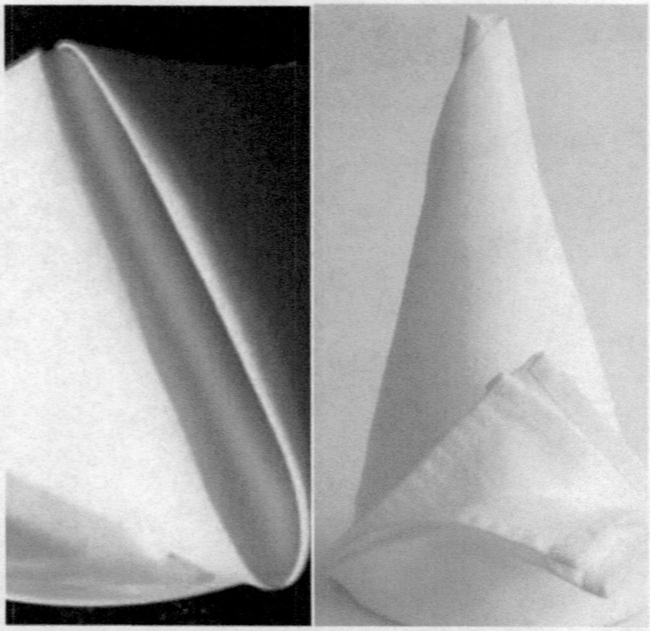

Pyramid fold, Clown fold

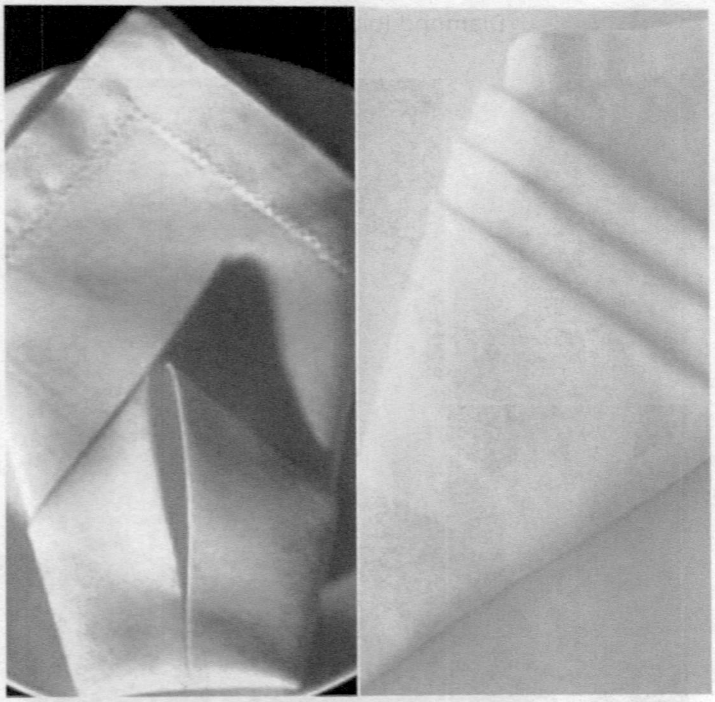

The cone fold

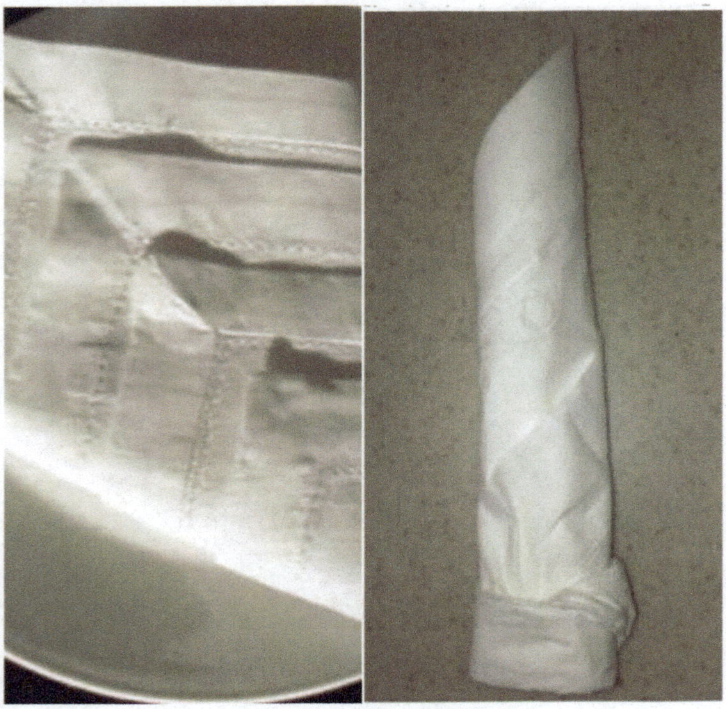

Diamond fold, candle fold

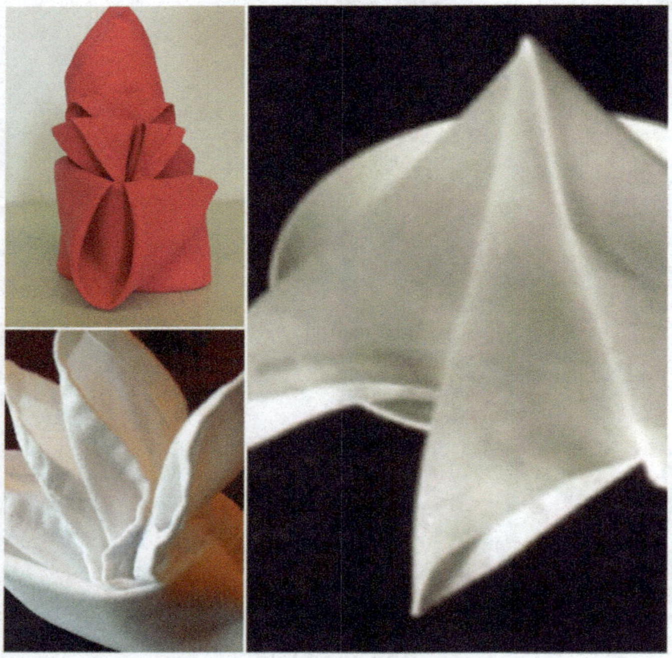

Arum fold, French fold, Bird of paradise fold.

HOTEL MANAGEMENT

TYPES OF COMMERCIAL LODGINGS

HOTEL:

A hotel is a commercial establishment offering lodging to travelers for short duration of time and sometimes to permanent residents, and often having restaurants, meeting rooms, stores, etc. that are available to the general public. It offers meals and other services. To be called a hotel it must have a minimum of six rooms and three must be attached to private bathroom facilities.

USA AND WORLDWIDE CLASSIFICATION OF HOTELS

1. **star *Moderate tourist.**
2. **star **Tourist class**
3. **star ***Superior tourists**
4. **star ****Moderate first class.**
5. **star *****Limited service first class**
6. **star ******First class**
7. **star ******* Moderate deluxe**
8. **star ********deluxe**
9. **star *********Superior deluxe**

MOTEL:

A motel is a hotel providing travelers with lodging and free parking facilities, typically a roadside hotel having rooms to the outside packing area or an urban hotel offering parking within the building. A combination of motorists (mot) and hotel (tel). Located on highways to allow travelers to spend the night and take rest for further traveling.

***INN*:**

A commercial establishment that provides lodging, food etc. for the public especially travelers, a small hotel, or a tavern.

GLOSSARY

1. Agbono. The seed of African mango use for cooking of soup. It can be an alternative to okro. It is also called bush mango, okwong or ndock chocolate.
2. Akob: The back of the garlic tree or African Davida. It is often called hyiomi, kanda stick or omiplat.
3. Akwa'a: Pounded cocoyams (Ngemba dialect.)
4. Akuuh: colocasia commonly called country cocoyam which is one of the cocoyam used for the achu foofoo.
5. Ambaa (Ambagü): Young cocoyam leaves used for preparing the black soup for achu.
6. Antwere: The blossom flower of the cocoyam plant. Also used to cook the black soup.
7. Anyéré: The African eggplant or garden egg
8. Ate: Young cocoyam leaves use for the achu soup.
9. Atii-tii: The black soup use for eating achu.
10. Atzhoh is seeds of heaven (Afromomium SP Uganda) often called Ndong, wild cardamom or Guinea pepper.
11. Awumne: A herb like spinach used in soups like okro soup and nkworo soup.
12. Ba'am is another name for huckleberry leaves
13. Bende is boiled cocoyam in Iroko language of Ndian Division.
14. Bewole is amaranth leaves
15. Bikwi is the traditional name for the African Black pepper or grains of selim (Xylopia aethiopica)

16. Bili – Bili (Bil-Bil) is a traditional drink made from millet.

17. Bilome: A Cameroonian spice for soup.

18. Bissap: Foléré, known as sorrel leaves or bissap.

19. Bongo long: Another name for Mbongo.

20. C.a.c : Cuillère à soupe (Tablespoon).

21. Chikwangues: Cassava batons (Bobolo and Miondo)

22. Chi Na'a: Achu soup with okro added. A specialty of the Bamileke ethnic group of Dschang.

23. Courgettes: Another name for zucchini, a vegetable similar to cucumber.

24. Dawa – dawa: seeds of the locust beans used as seasoning in soups. (Parkia biglobosa)

25. Dibanga: another name for crayfish (small, dried shrimps)

26. Dibaka: one of two thiny miondo strips tied together

27. Ecorce rouge (Hiomi) Bark of tree grated and used as a spice. (Hypodophnis zenkeri) Nkouppo.

28. Ecrevisse: French name for crayfish

29. Erembi: cocoyam leaves

30. Eseke- seke: Aridan seed (Tetrapleura tetraptera) a spice used in many Cameroonian soups. Commonly called 3-side.

31. Essouk: A Beti name for mbanga soup.

32. Feuille d'airelles: Huckleberry leaves.

33. Feuille d'Odzom: Ginger-type leaves used as a spice. A bay leave can replace the ginger leaves

34. Fii: Ngemba name for amaranth.

35. Folon: A Beti name for amaranth.

36. Foulom: A Ngemba name for a Cameroon spice often called country onion (Afrostyrax lepidopyhllus) Also called oignon sauvage.

37. Fünüsongnü: Young shoots of the elephant grass used as a vegetable.

38. Gateau: French name for cake

39. Graine de courge: Melon seeds

40. Gourd seed: Calabash egusi of green pumpkin seeds.

41. Herbs odorants: Perfumed spices.

42. Kanwa: Limestone used to emulsify achu soup and to maintain the green color of vegetables. Also called Akanwa.

43. Katanga: It is the skin of cattle cooked as meat in some Cameroonian soups.

44. Katti – katti: It is open-fire roasted chopped chicken in palm oil and seasoning, usually only salt.

45. Keleng – keleng: The traditional name for jute mallow. It's a glutinous vegetable. Also called cren-cren.

46. Kieng: A Ngemba name for one of the spices of achu soup (Xylopia aethiopic). It is also called grains of selim, Senegal pepper and Bikwi.

47. Kilichl: A special spiced beef, dried in the sun and grilled.

48. Kossam: A name for Cameroon yoghurt

49. Kotmargin (cutmargin). Its African basil. Also called L'ossim Nnam in Beti. (Ocimum gratissimum)

50. Kwacha: A traditional drink made from corn.

51. Jollof muscle: The dish is said to have originated from Senegal, where Jollof is a Wolof word meaning “one pot” but it is also poular in countries like Gambia.

52. Lalo: A name for the jute mallow (cren-cren), keleng- keleng by the people of the North part of Cameroon.

53. Oseille: Sorrel leaves also called Bissap.

54. Macab: It is macabo (Xanthosoma sagittifolium)

55. Makere: Boiled plantains

56. Masala: A Lesotho spice

57. Masepo, Massep: Its wild basil

58. Matangaa: Pink colocasia esculenta.

59. Makpamba (cassava tuber)

60. Mbanga: Palm nuts.

61. Mbongo: African spice (Bastered Melengueta,) Afromomium danielli and Afromomium citrantum. Also known as Bongo long, Vongolo and Tchouoko

62. Melon seeds: White egusi or country egusi

63. Medjanga: Crayfish

64. Minde: Cocoyam leaves

65. Mpah: Spinach – like herbs used in glutinous soup. Also called Awumne.

66. Ndzaa, Njaa name for soup in Ngemba and bafut

67. Nding: African nutmeg. (Pébè)

68. Ndong: Seed of heaven (Afromomium SP Uganda)

69. Nikii: Locally made limestone with woodash or green plantain peelings.

70. Nwi, Nkworo, Nku: A glutinous soup

71. Njama – njama: Huckleberry leaves. Also called night shade.

72. Ngon: Egusi in Bulu and Ewondo

73. Ngondo: Groundnuts in Bakweri

74. Nnam Owondo: Beti name for groundnut paste.

75. Okongobong: Leaves of a pumpkin gourd with a fluted shape used for soups.

76. Pébè: African or Calabash nutmeg (Mondora myristica)

77. Pili – pili: Bird's eye pepper, Tita Sing in Ngemba, Chili pepper or Thai pepper. (Petit piment)

78. Shaah: A drink brewed from fermented corn.

79. Sopp: A Ngemba name for a West African pepper, called Jowe, uziza pepper a main spice of achu soup (Piper guineese)

80. Sougi: Mbanga soup by the Bassa group

81. Timba Na Busa: sese equacoco in mbanga soup.

82. Uboh: Ngemba name for mushroom. Locally called Kokobiako.

83. Wolanga: Mamie Cocoyam pounded foofoo.

84. Welolo: Mbonga or Herring fish

85. Wosangu: Huckleberry leaves in Bakweri

86. Waghu: Blackeye pea leaves used as vegetables in Ngemba.

87. Zom: Huckleberry leaves in Beti

BIBLOGRAPHY

Abigael Djeumen: Les Delices de la cuisine Camerounaise Tome 1

Abigael Djeumen: Les Delices de la cuisine Camerounaise Nouveau

Abigael Djeumen: Jus Boisson et Salads de Fruits, Naturels.

Anita Tull: Food & Nutrition, Oxford, 1996.

Basic Restaurant Training Manual.

Cameroon Tourism Guide: Wala Edition. January 2002 edition

Che Gustav N/Mbinka Aloysia/Nkeinen Celestine/Sante B: Cullinary Recipe Book for "O" & "A" Levels.

Enid O' Reilly – Wright: The Student Cookery Book, Oxford, 1994

Family Favorites Cookbook, 1979

Gwen Mckee and Barbara Moseley: Best of the Best from IOWA. Selected Recipes from Iowa's Favorite Cookbooks. 1997

Jeanne Chatelier Délices des Bons Petits Plats

Jordan S. Rubin: The Maker's Diet: 2004.

Jo Ann Shirley: Wonderful ways to prepare Hors D'oeuvres & First courses

K.E. Idowu: Aunti Kate's Cookery Book, 1985

K.E. Idowu: Les Bonne Recettes de Tante Cathy, 1986

Les classiques Africains # 921. La cuisine aux pays de soleil, 1976

Les classiques Africains # 908 Hygiene Alimentaire, 1977

M. Fabien Bellahsen, M. Andre Delmoral: Délices de la Cuisine Créole.

Michel Chapelier, Jean Charles Tsokona Yanzeu, Pascal Gbikpi: Le soja Recette de cuisine au soja au soja First Edition, 1984

Nathaniel Okenyi Eyong-Echaw: Advanced Level Food Science and Nutrition. 2013

Phebe N. Ndam. A safari of choice African Cuisine. First Edition 198

Sr. Marie Chantal Asom: Basic knowledge in Home Economics.

Ta kemore Chagomoka, Regine Kamga, Abdou, Tenkouano, Maureen Mocozzi: Traditional Vegetables Recipes from Cameroon, Amaranth, African Eggplant, Jute Mallow, Nightshades and Okra, 2014

24.The Australian Women's weekly. Barbecue. Fast recipes using Take away chicken

ABOUT THE AUTHOR

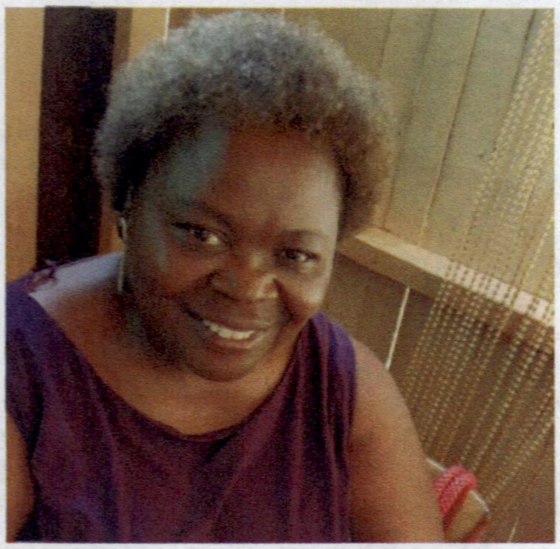

BI CHIBIKOM THERESIA NIBA was born in Mankon, Bamenda. She attended the Girl's Primary School Big Mankon and the Catholic Primary School Ntambeng Mankon before proceeding to the St Pius X Teacher training college Tatum, Nso in Bui Division, Cameroon in 1968. She had the Teachers' Grade 11 certificate, the Ordinary and Advanced Level Certificates between 1973-1975.

In 1976 she was admitted into the University of Arkansas, at Fayetteville, United States of America where she specialized and graduated with a Bachelor of Science degree in Home economics education in 1980. Upon her return to Cameroon in 1981 she joined the Cameroon Public Service as a Home Economics teacher. She taught in various secondary and Technical colleges, both private and with the Government in Cameroon. In addition to her teaching career, she has been actively involved in many courses for family life enrichment and personality development.

She is a trained catechist from the Higher Institute of Religious studies, Maryvale Institute Bamenda. She retired from active service in 2013 and she is actively involved in Catechesis, Parish based activities, Catering, Home making, writing and private business. In addition to parish documents she has written the biography of her beloved father Tata Maximus Chi-Bikom Mukunglla II in 2015.

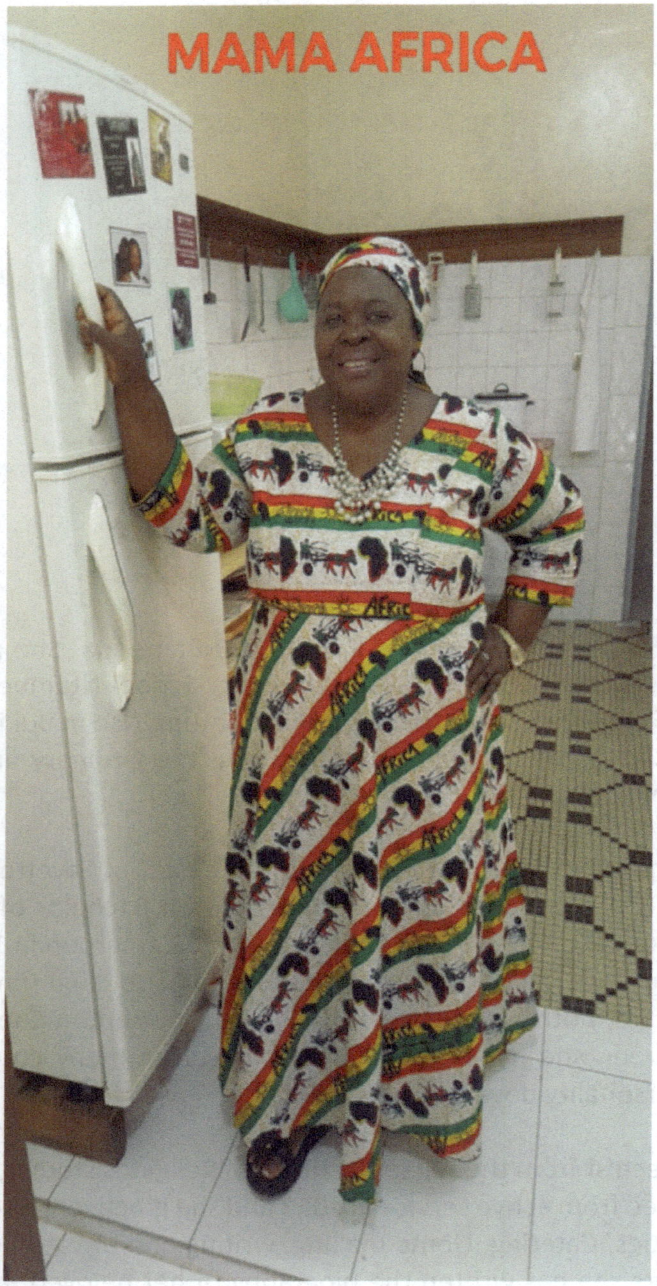
MAMA AFRICA

Made in United States
North Haven, CT
18 October 2026

20554115R00161